Thinking
A·I·D·S

**ADDISON-WESLEY
PUBLISHING COMPANY, INC.**

Reading, Massachusetts   Menlo Park, California

New York   Don Mills, Ontario

Wokingham, England   Amsterdam   Bonn

Sydney   Singapore   Tokyo   Madrid   San Juan

Thinking
A·I·D·S

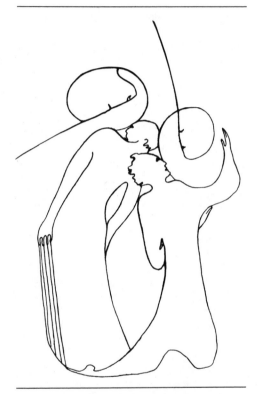

MARY CATHERINE
BATESON

AND RICHARD
GOLDSBY

Many of the designations used by manufacturers and sellers
to distinguish their products are claimed as trademarks.
Where those designations appear in this book and Addison-
Wesley was aware of a trademark claim, the designations
have been printed in initial capital letters (i.e., Krazy
Glue).

Library of Congress Cataloging-in-Publication Data

Bateson, Mary Catherine.
    Thinking AIDS / Mary Catherine Bateson and Richard
      Goldsby.
        p.   cm.
      Bibliography: p. 162–165.
      Includes index.
      ISBN 0-201-15594-X
      ISBN 0-201-19579-8 (pbk.)
        1. AIDS (Disease)—Social aspects.   2. AIDS (Disease)—
Psychological aspects.   I. Goldsby, Richard A. II. Title.
RA644.A25B37   1988
362.1'9697'92—dc19   88-14599

Jacket and text design by Copenhaver Cumpston
Jacket and title page illustration: *La Manos* (or) *Conversations
avec l'autre monde*, ca. 1930 by Romaine Brooks. Pencil and
chalk on paper, 18½ × 12³⁄₁₆″. Reproduced courtesy Na-
tional Museum of American Art, Smithsonian Institution.
Gift of the artist.
Set in 11½ point Garamond no. 3 by DEKR Corporation,
Woburn, MA

ABCDEFGHIJ-HA-89
First printing, July 1988
First paperback edition, June 1989

In appreciation of teachers, who can make all the difference in giving young people a sense of what they can be and do,

we dedicate this book to two teachers from our high school days,

Luke Ponder

for his work with the Redaels at Lincoln High School in Kansas City,

and

Josephine Hornor Belknap

for her teaching of mathematics at the Brearley School in New York.

■

No man is an island, entire of itself; every man
is a piece of the continent, a part of the main;
if a clod be washed away by the sea, Europe is
the less, as well as if a promontory were, as
well as if a manor of thy friends or of thine
own were; any man's death diminishes me,
because I am involved in mankind; and
therefore never send to know for whom
the bell tolls; it tolls for thee.

JOHN DONNE

DEVOTIONS UPON
EMERGENT OCCASIONS, 1624, NO. 17.

CONTENTS

■

ACKNOWLEDGMENTS

■

THE AUTHORS met at Amherst College in 1982, which demonstrates that small liberal arts colleges can provide the setting for interdisciplinary conversation as well as campus politics. Each of us has benefited from a number of other relationships and institutional ties in our work together.

Mary Catherine Bateson wishes to acknowledge the support of the Guggenheim Foundation during 1987–88, primarily granted for a concurrent project on modalities of commitment in women's lives. For a first opportunity to think about the scientific context of AIDS she wishes to thank the Rockefeller Foundation, which sponsored a conference on "Subviral Pathogens of Plants and Animals: Viroids and Prions" while she was a resident scholar at their Bellagio Study and Conference Center in the summer of 1983. Since May 1987 she has been a member of a series of conferences organized by Stewart Brand and supported by Shell, Volvo, and AT&T to explore the theme of organizational learning, which took the AIDS epidemic as a study topic; a great deal of useful material was circulated in this group, and she is especially indebted to it for analyses by Francisco Varela and Kees van der Heijden and for the opportunity to participate in ongoing computer conferencing while writing.

Richard Goldsby wishes to thank Thomas Kindt for a sabbatic year spent in 1981 at his Laboratory of Immunogenetics at the National Institutes of Health where he first learned about AIDS; the Department of Animal Science at the University of Massachusetts, Amherst; and Theodore Cross, who made his work at Amherst College possible.

We have both benefited immeasurably from the critiques and suggestions of friends, including Ellen Bassuk, Fred Feldman, José Girón, Richard Godsey, G. Evelyn Hutchinson, and Thomas Kindt, and of our agent, John Brockman, and our editor, Jane Isay. We are also grateful for assistance from the ever helpful academic computer facility and library of Amherst College. Our spouses, Barbara Osborne and J. Barkev Kassarjian, have given every kind of practical and intellectual support.

We would probably not have undertaken this project except for the AIDS victims we have known, and want particularly to remember here William Whitehead and Tom Waddell. The memory of human and intellectual quality they represent has been a constant reminder of the epidemic's toll.

A NOTE ON
TERMINOLOGY

■

THE TERM "AIDS" is an acronym for Acquired Immune
Deficiency Syndrome that has rapidly become a word in
its own right and taken on two inconsistent meanings.
As used and clinically defined by the medical profession,
it refers to a group of conditions developing in the state
of immune system collapse caused by infection with one
of the Human Immunodeficiency Viruses (HIV). So far,
clinical AIDS is always a terminal state. "AIDS," however, has come to be used much more broadly to refer
to the entire range of phenomena associated with HIV
infection. In this discussion we follow this colloquial
usage, which is probably irreversible, and use the term
"full-blown AIDS" for the medically defined syndrome.
There has also been confusion about the name of the
virus, but after a variety of conflicting namings, HIV
has become the accepted technical term and will be used
here in alternation with the term "AIDS virus."

Thinking
A·I·D·S

1

INTRODUCTION

∎

A PREVIOUSLY UNKNOWN life form, the virus that causes AIDS, is now making its way through the human population, spreading around the world with devastating and accelerating effects. That virus has become a part of the biological context of our lives, one of the many life forms that actually live inside of human beings rather than around them. All of these can potentially be known and at least partially controlled but the needed thinking about AIDS has just begun, and it is already clear that it raises the most basic questions about the human condition, about human biology, and about the mechanisms of social life.

The AIDS epidemic, as it moves around the planet, is posing new questions about justice and teaching us new ways of thinking about human learning and human suffering. It throws certain characteristics of society into sharp relief, just as radioisotopes, moving through the body, can be used to highlight physiological processes for diagnosis. At one level the movement of the epidemic reflects communication and travel. At another it belies our habitual self-deceptions, tracing activities that would otherwise be secret: drug addiction and sexual practices that most people have preferred not to know about—extramarital sex, homosexuality, prostitution. AIDS has made us newly aware of human diversity. In our own society it forces us to acknowledge bisexuality, a pattern of sexual preference that most Americans, who like their distinctions clear, have tended to ignore, and is making us more aware of middle-class intravenous drug use. It will probably increase awareness of the sexual use of children, of sex in prisons, of sex and drugs in the peacetime army.

AIDS highlights processes of social change: urbanization and monetary economies in Africa that send men to the cities for cash earnings while their wives stay in the villages to farm; changed sexual mores for heterosexuals as well as homosexuals; the economic dislocations and prejudice that are increasingly turning some minority communities in America into an underclass. The history of failure to heed the early warnings of the epidemic is a statement of our priorities as a society. Now that we know how to prevent the disease from spreading, its continued spread must advertise the ways in which, in this interconnected and interdependent world, we fail to communicate to individuals the very knowledge they need to survive. AIDS moves along the fault lines of our society and becomes a metaphor for understanding that society.

The process of learning how to think about and control AIDS is a step in human evolution, for the application of knowledge is the distinctive evolutionary mechanism of our species. Human beings adapt to their environments not primarily through biological evolution, which works rather slowly, but through cultural evolution, changes in shared knowledge expressed in changes in behavior. We know the history of many of these changes and know that culture makes human beings more rapidly and flexibly adaptable than any other species. We know too that the AIDS epidemic is not the first occasion when the biological context of human life has changed dangerously, nor will it be the last. Still, as the AIDS epidemic tests our understanding of social and cultural mechanisms, it reveals in us a curious kind of helplessness in moving from information to changes in behavior.

It is not easy to think about AIDS. Most of us react with a mixture of sympathy and horror to the personal tragedies we read about or encounter, yet in order to think about AIDS we need to illuminate the emotions that the disease inspires with a new kind of cross-section of human knowledge.

AIDS proposes questions of the highest human and intellectual importance. The biology of AIDS lies right at the cutting edge of research. We live in an age when the biological sciences are reaching for the kind of power and clarity that has characterized physics; like physics, this new thrust of knowledge presents both possibilities and dangers. Some of humankind's greatest achievements have involved the effort to control biological phenomena, often only half knowing what we were doing and why. Many of the greatest of these achievements lie in the ancient past: the abilities to shape life forms to our purposes by domesticating plants and animals and even microorganisms like yeast, as well as the ability to defend ourselves against others. The potential of modern biology arises from the development of techniques that permit inspection of the finest grain of physical and biological processes so that the properties and behavior of living things begin to be explicable in terms of the physical structure of molecules. At the same time, questions remain about how these intricate processes are integrated in living wholes.

Viruses are the smallest forms to which we attribute life, and indeed can barely be called living, so whoever would understand the nature of life must be interested in the viruses, right at that crucial threshold. Viruses are not autonomously capable of many of the functions of cells, but they do carry genetic information. To fulfill these missing functions, they must gain admission to cells and inhabit them. Because the AIDS virus selectively invades the cells of the immune system, virology opens into immunology, the science that studies the maintenance of identity within the organism and its internal interactions with other forms of life.

Immunology focuses on the relationship between what happens at levels smaller than the cell—at the molecular level—and the fate of the whole organism. It may eventually provide the intellectual bridge between these different visions. But AIDS also challenges a look at populations and at ecological interactions. Questions about how a biological process like the spread of an epidemic affects a population take us right into contemporary understandings of evolution, where we now know that we have to look at populations in environments rather than at single organisms.

An understanding of the AIDS epidemic and how it can be controlled requires understanding of the development of shared knowledge and behavior patterns, particularly at the interface between biology and the learned characteristics of human communities, like language or purposeful invention or the effort to find meaning in natural events. These are anthropological issues, but AIDS forces us to pose questions in every one of the social sciences and reveals the limitations of our applicable knowledge at every turn. It drives us to psychology, with questions about how individuals learn and change their behavior; to sociology, to understand change and the processes of inclusion and exclusion in large groups and institutions; to economics, to understand the effect of such changes on the use of resources; and to political science and ethics, to understand the processes of decision making when the needs and desires of individuals are weighed against those of the larger society. In order to think about the AIDS epidemic and how it affects the future of our species, all of these different ways of looking at the lives of individuals and communities must be woven together, at one moment emphasizing their commonalities, at another the distinctive features of each.

Human attention is profoundly shaped by love and danger and early death. Diseases and the social responses to them have been critical in human history, and have been explored by artists and philosophers as well as scientists, wondering about issues of good and evil and how these are connected to the mysteries of death and suffering. We have been speaking here of understanding as if it were an analytical process, but analysis is only one step toward understanding. Every generation must integrate knowledge and experience, finding them meaningful or absurd, tempted by distortions and self-deception when they seem to make our world more coherent. Many who have written about the AIDS epidemic have written out of an urgent need to convey the depth of suffering involved and to evoke compassion from a society that appeared unfeeling. We have chosen here to put less emphasis on the horrors of full-blown AIDS and more emphasis on social adaptations to controlling the virus that causes it, for we write out of the conviction that horror is not the best place to begin in constructing individual and social change. Horror creates the impulse to denial. Instead, we are concerned with presenting the AIDS epidemic as a fact of the world in which we now live and with demonstrating that, by responding generously and wisely, we can make our society a better one, enriching our living and our dying.

Of all the literature of illness, the work that most poignantly evokes the tension between cultural meaning and individual suffering is the biblical Book of Job. Job has always been virtuous, public-spirited, and wealthy, when suddenly everything begins to go wrong. His children are killed, his money is lost, and his skin breaks out in boils from head to toe. He longs for death and wishes he had never been born. He gets scant comfort from his friends, who gather to argue that he must have deserved his sufferings at the hand of God, that divine justice must be apparent in the events of this life. Job adamantly denies that he has done anything to deserve his afflictions and longs to argue his case with God: "Though he slay me, yet will I trust in him: but I will maintain my own ways before him" (13:15).

After many chapters of self-righteous sermonizing by Job's "friends," God himself speaks from a whirlwind and says, with a wealth of examples from natural history, it is all much more complicated than you know, you cannot claim to understand my ways. A vision of the intricacy of the natural world is offered that is not organized around human needs but that frames the lives and interlocking needs of all the wild creatures of the forests and mountains, eagles and lions and mountain goats, and the leviathan in the depths of the sea.

> Doth the eagle mount up at thy command,
>   and make her nest on high?

> She dwelleth and abideth on the rock,
>   upon the crag of the rock, and the strong
>   place.

> From thence she seeketh the prey,
>   and her eyes behold afar off.

> Her young ones also suck up blood:
>   and where the slain are, there is she.

> (JOB 39:27–30)

Job is silenced, saying, "I have uttered that I understood not, things too wonderful for me, which I knew not" (42:3). His concern with his own affairs and with human definitions of virtue is put into a wider perspective. The gift of wonder assuages his loss.

We know today a great deal about the interlocking lives of different species. We know that to begin to understand the survival of any species requires painstaking observation and detailed knowledge of the environment, and we have learned, at least to some degree, the poet's concern for what goes on invisible to us, in sea or wilderness or on a scale too small for our vision. But we still slip into seeing these matters from the human point of view, turning knowledge of the natural world into parables of divine justice and human mastery. The equivalent today of the lesson in natural history that God gave to Job might be the depiction of the extraordinary elegance and complexity of the finest grain of natural phenomena, the microscopic dramas and adaptations of other organisms, including the AIDS virus that makes its nest and brings forth its young within the human immune system itself. The widened perspective that Job is given might today include other human ways in other times and places, ways of surviving and finding pleasure far outside the Hebrew imagination of right and wrong. But of course Job's comforters are engaged in "saving God," which means hanging on to a way of thinking about the universe that makes sense to them.

The habits of thought that made Job's comforters so ready to condemn him are still with us. Persons afflicted with AIDS lose first their health, then many of their friends and family and resources, then their lives. Unlike Job, many people with AIDS were poor or rejected before they became ill, but the illness will affect rich and poor alike. Many must acknowledge that they have behaved in ways that their neighbors regard as immoral, and may concur in that blame. Many people with AIDS suffer an additional burden of guilt for probably having passed the disease to others.

Nevertheless, the spread of AIDS to the newborn and the horrors of its clinical course are for many sufficient refutation of the argument that it could represent divine justice. The proportion of AIDS patients who are like Job in living highly conventional lives is increasing steadily. More and more spouses who are neither drug-addicted nor promiscuous are contracting AIDS from their partners, more and more infants are being born carrying their deaths within them. Until the mid-1980s, the AIDS virus was being sown through American and European populations with blood products, and medical transmission is still significant in third world countries. Furthermore, many behaviors that transmit AIDS, even if they might have been condemned in terms of conventional moralities, are now widely shared: not only are almost half of all American teenagers sexually active by the end of high school, but the candidates for the U.S. presidential nomination for 1988 included two ministers whose children were conceived well before marriage.

Almost everyone can find something to disapprove of in the behavior of some AIDS patients. Job's comforters argue that all humans share in guilt, so perhaps from that perspective even Job's children deserved their deaths. But disapproval quickly becomes an obstacle to understanding.

The most dangerous thing about self-righteousness is the inference made by those who regard themselves as virtuous that they are different and therefore safe, and that if the disease progresses unchecked, society will be purged while they remain untouched. Not us—them. This attitude was a major block to organizing and funding the medical research needed to deal with the emergency, and continues to hinder efforts to protect and care for those threatened by the disease.

The alternative position is one of empathy and the acknowledgment by the society at large that those who are suffering from AIDS are very much like themselves. Indeed, dealing with the epidemic requires looking at themselves and at the epidemic with new eyes. This understanding requires the insight that people of color are like white people, that rich people are like poor, and that the destinies of people on every continent are woven together. We are defined as a single species by the capacity for interbreeding, and human beings everywhere cross lines of class and race in the search for sexual partners, sometimes in tenderness and other times in exploitation. Epidemiologists must speak in terms of risk groups to explain the development of epidemics, but unlike some diseases whose risk groups are clearly bounded by genetics or geography, the ultimate risk group for AIDS includes every human being.

The appropriate responses to the AIDS epidemic are

both social and personal. They are late in coming and it is already clear that the costs of delay will be heavy. It takes genuine emotional involvement to decide to change one's lifestyle and take precautions against AIDS, real concern for oneself or loved ones. It also takes informed understanding and information. When the threat still seems to be at a distance, such changes require deeply felt imaginative identification, and it is the lack of this act of the imagination that keeps people with a full intellectual understanding of the danger from taking action. Unfortunately, infection has tended to spread faster than either empathic emotional involvement or understanding. Fear has proved sufficient to trigger prejudice more quickly than behavioral change, because prejudice creates emotional distance, putting the danger at arm's length.

The AIDS epidemic will cost us dearly. Perhaps we will gain wisdom from it, not only in the fields of virology and biochemistry but also in an understanding of the social costs of exclusion and despair. From a concern for the immune systems of individuals we will have to move to an understanding of the immune systems of societies, the patterns of vigilance and caring that protect their continuing health. The same forces that make it hard to use the biology-culture relationship to address AIDS face every effort to discover distinctively human solutions—the solutions of intelligence and choice, of discipline and imagination—to the problems of the modern world.

In the years ahead, the awareness of AIDS will resonate in visions as well as nightmares, providing the stuff of art and the echoes of revelation, as well as opening new doors of scientific understanding. The AIDS crisis represents an immense tragedy for many persons and a danger for many more. It also represents an opportunity for changes in our understanding of human biology and social life and the ways in which we use knowledge. From this point of view, the epidemic is a moment of opportunity for discovering the full potential of humanness. If we can use the impetus of AIDS to expand and apply knowledge cooperatively and humanely, we may also learn to control the dangers of the arms race and of world hunger and environmental degradation, for the imagination of AIDS is the imagination of human unity, intimately held in the interdependent web of life.

2

THE ECOLOGIES

OF DISEASE

■

LIFE ON THIS PLANET involves interactions among a very large and diverse range of organisms which depend on one another in a great many different ways. When we think of human dependence on other life forms, the tendency is to think first of the plants and animals we use for food or fiber. It takes a moment to remember that the atmosphere of the planet—the air we breathe— is the joint product of the life processes of plants, animals, and microorganisms; that the soil from which plants grow is necessarily teeming with organic life; and that the human body itself supports an ongoing population of microorganisms. The environment in which any given organism flourishes is always a community of interacting life forms. This is equally true of the bacteria living in the intestine and of the squirrels in an oak forest.

One of the central concepts of modern ecology is that of the *niche*. A niche involves not only location but also behavior; it is a behavioral space in which an organism moves and competes for resources. Many species coexist in a forest, but each one can be seen to have a slightly different niche. Woodpeckers drilling into trees to find insects boring inside are usually not in competition with squirrels gathering acorns or even with the many other bird species gathering seeds or capturing other kinds of insects. The system of niches orchestrates the encounters and separations of the myriad species in the forest.

Human beings living in a city are similar, for just as a bird or a beetle interacts selectively with different parts of the life of a forest, so different people live differently in a city. For one person—call her Ms. Parker—New York is a gigantic parking problem, but she may never use public transport; for another, whom we recognize as Mr. Rider, the subways are essential to day-to-day life, and he experiences the street grid in terms of the location of stations, reads subway ads, and worries about being mugged. Some individuals encounter each other for help and harm as they move between home and work and recreation; others, even in a small geographical space, might almost be on different planets. You can think of these different individuals as living in different behavioral niches within the city: the way you use and interact with your environment *is* your environment. In the example given here, it is easy to imagine changes that affect the behavioral space of our two individuals, Parker and Rider, bringing them into competition for the same resources or forcing one of them to leave the city. The parking regulations may change and Parker may ride. The public transport workers may go on strike and Rider may buy a car. They may meet each other on foot or get jobs in the same office. Technology may offer a new option—a splendid new form of moped—that both of them want, and they may be in competition for service.

Since the appearance of Homo sapiens, the way humans use and affect their environment has changed steadily, altering the niches of all other forms of life, sometimes drastically enough to cause extinction. Human behavioral changes are particularly important for understanding diseases that involve interactions between humans and other life forms, those diseases in which the human body is the natural habitat for some other organism during all or part of its life cycle. Many pathogens live in a stable relationship with a human population, but that relationship may be disrupted by advances in public health or medicine. Worldwide vaccination programs denied to the smallpox virus the only environment in which it could live and reproduce, so it is believed to be extinct. Sometimes a pathogen will suddenly multiply when some environmental change, caused by custom or technology, gives it the chance radically to expand its niche. On the other hand, species that destroy their own environments cannot themselves survive. This has implications for human behavior as well as for understanding the mechanisms of diseases in which one organism lives in the body of another.

It is possible for an epidemic to arise rapidly from a random genetic change or mutation, but that mutation must occur in an environment in which the new form has a selective advantage. Otherwise, new genetic variations may survive but be practically invisible. Any wild species has a great deal of naturally occurring genetic variation. The reservoir of genetic variation is what allows a species to survive when some environmental circumstance wipes out most of its members. What is important to notice here is that epidemics are created by a combination of genetic potential and environmental opportunity.

It will be helpful, in thinking about the AIDS epidemic, to remember that pathogens—life forms that inhabit other life forms and in doing so cause disease—face the same problems of adaptation and survival as other kinds of organisms. There is no way to locate with certainty the original genetic events that bring a disease into being. It may eventually be shown that the pathogen has existed for a long time in a different niche, for example, in another species, like one of our primate relatives; but if it arose from a recent mutation or a series of relatively recent genetic changes, whether in a human being or in some other species, it may prove extremely difficult to establish the exact time and place of those events. In any case, the important question about any newly recognized disease is the niche in which it now propagates. Is this niche one that we have created? Is it one that we have the capacity to control and reshape? Why is this particular life form proving successful enough to reproduce and spread widely? How does the survival strategy of a particular pathogen resemble other diseases? These are the ecological questions we should be asking about the AIDS virus.

Epidemics of plague have recurred through human history with such devastating effect that the name of a particular disease caused by *Yersinia pestis* is synonymous with the concept of a catastrophic epidemic. *Y. pestis* is an ovoid bacterium* that lives and breeds in the digestive tract of several species of flea that make their home on rodents, drinking their blood. The bacteria are tolerable to the flea, but they do present a mild problem when they proliferate, solved when the flea regurgitates into the rat at the time of a blood meal. The bacteria then continue to live and proliferate in the bloodstream of the rat, so that other fleas, drawing blood from the same rat, also become carriers. For the rat, however, the bacteria are likely to be fatal, as they become fully virulent only at mammalian body temperatures. When the rat dies, its resident population of fleas, infected with the bacteria, go in search of alternative hosts.

When the life cycle of a pathogen depends on mobility provided by another species, often without damage, the carrier species is called a *vector*. The fleas prefer rodent hosts, so the natural life cycle of *Y. pestis* involves transitions from rodent to flea to rodent. When this natural cycle is altered, the possibility of epidemic arises, but plague exists around us today, without triggering human epidemics, among wild rodents such as prairie dogs that

---

* The familiar terminology for different types of bacteria (bacillus, spirochete, and so on) is based on shape as seen through the microscope. We have preferred to emphasize the common characteristics of all bacterial pathogens and to use the more general terminology for all.

have naturally developed immunity. Under most circumstances a human host is unlikely to be a handy alternative for a flea departing from a dead prairie dog, but this is a reason for caution in handling the bodies of dead wild animals. Fortunately, fleas are conservative creatures: each kind of flea has its preferred hosts and doesn't switch hosts when it is doing well.

The great plagues of medieval Europe were caused by changes in human behavior. The first and most important changes represented a vast opportunity for rats. The city has been an important human invention and can be regarded from the human point of view as the niche in which civilization developed, but the aggregation of large numbers of human beings, with their garbage and bodily wastes, created ecological niches for many other species including rats, cockroaches, and starlings. The second class of changes created links between reservoirs of infection, for as human beings traveled for trade and exploration, they carried with them rats, rat fleas, and human fleas. The Middle Ages were a very itchy time, with fleas and bedbugs everywhere. Interestingly, several of the measures taken by human beings to protect themselves actually spread the danger: the burning of buildings occupied by plague victims drove out the infected rats in their foundations, and the flight of those who had contracted the disease but did not yet show symptoms carried it to new towns and countries, where it was passed from human to human, even in the absence of rats, by human fleas.

Like most bacterial diseases, plague can be treated with the appropriate antibiotic, and natural immunity exists among some humans and rodents, especially those who have survived previous infection. The prevention of plague depends, however, on neutralizing the effects of behaviors that create reservoirs of rats and fleas and that link them to each other. A sudden attack on rodent populations could trigger an epidemic by letting loose large numbers of homeless rat fleas, but long-term sustained rodent control, achieved by good sanitation and garbage disposal, largely eliminates alternative carriers. Hawsers—large ropes that attach ships to docks when they are in port—have metal disks on them to control hitchhiking rats, and cases of plague are closely monitored worldwide. Plague epidemics have killed millions of people and unguessable millions of rats, but today, although all the species concerned continue to exist in many places, there are only a handful of cases every year. The behavioral changes that controlled plague were largely public and carried other more immediately obvious benefits: less itching, fewer piles of garbage. Fortunately, it was not necessary to attack the problem of plague by giving up travel or urban living.

A number of diseases are sexually transmitted from person to person, and although their life cycles and effects within the body vary, they often co-occur in the same patient. Syphilis is a bacterial disease with an ecology closely analogous to that of AIDS, and was regarded with similar fear and horror before the discovery of penicillin. Syphilis lives its entire life cycle inside human beings and kills slowly. This allows plenty of time for the infection to be transmitted from host to host. When syphilis emerged in Europe at the end of the fifteenth century, its spread, like that of so many venereal diseases, was hastened by factors that separated men from their families, especially warfare. It was at first extremely virulent but over time became less so, perhaps because those strains that gave the host more time to propagate the disease were more successful; syphilis still remains endemic all over the world.

At one time the problem of sexually transmitted diseases (STDs) seemed essentially under control, but in recent decades, with changing sexual practices and the increased importance of several viruses, the landscape has changed. Another STD, gonorrhea, provides an interesting example of how a pathogen can evolve as a result of a selective pressure created by medication. It was at one time possible to prevent gonorrhea by administering sulfonamides, for instance, to all military recruits, but this allowed for the emergence of resistant strains. Fortunately, gonorrhea could still be treated with penicillin, but penicillin-resistant strains have also been developing.

Sometimes a change in technology creates a new niche in which a widespread but barely noticed organism can flourish dangerously. In 1976 delegates returning home from an American Legion Convention in Philadelphia started dying from a previously unknown bacterium which was later identified and named and shown to be relatively common. Human arrangements had created an ideal new niche for *Legionella* in the recirculating air-conditioning system of a hotel, where the bacteria multiplied and then were wafted into the lungs of the legionnaires. Similarly, in toxic shock syndrome, changes in tampon technology created an environment for local bacterial runaway. In both of these cases, changes in human behavior allowed for local rapid growth of bacteria but not for geographical spread. The sites where ambitious pathogens were multiplying were not interconnected, and the circumstances that promoted rapid growth could be eliminated.

At the opposite extreme, diseases like flu or the common cold pass easily and directly from person to person through the inhalation of virus-containing droplets. They in turn sometimes have the effect of creating vulnerability to other diseases such as pneumonia, so that influenza can be seen as an important part of the ecology of *Pneumococcus*, as a co-factor creating the conditions in which it in turn can flourish. The niches of influenza and cold viruses are shaped by travel and by social practices leading to concentrations of people, including nursery school children—but limiting such contact would be more burdensome than the disease.

One last example of environmental change may be useful: schistosomiasis. This debilitating disease is caused by flatworms that live a portion of the life cycle inside the human body and a portion in the bodies of a species of snail. In between, the larvae swim freely, seeking their next host. There is a loop here—humans, to water, to snails, to water, and back to humans—that can be cut at several different points, and attempts to control the disease often cut into the cycle more then once. It is possible to prevent larvae from passing from infected humans to water, since like many diseases they make this transition in the feces and can be prevented by hygienic disposal of human wastes. It is possible to reduce the availability of standing bodies of water or to attack the snails. And it is possible to prevent the parasites' transition from water back into the human body by wearing boots, though governments usually find it easier to apply snail-control chemicals to pools than to persuade peasants working in rice paddies to change their work habits, avoiding exposure of the skin to infested water. The least effective form of control is the treatment of infected individuals, which is expensive and physically traumatic.

Human beings have frequently enlarged the niche of schistosomes by creating year-round bodies of water for irrigation, most notably the Aswan High Dam in Egypt. Another source of spread in some places is the pool that traditionally stands outside every mosque to provide for ritual ablutions before prayer. Thus the niche in which the flatworms live is shaped both by agricultural practice and by religious belief. In other cases, like trichinosis, religious regulations about behavior have a protective effect.

The virus that causes AIDS is probably rather new, and may differ only minutely from some less successful precursor. There are tantalizing hints, for instance, of cases of an immune deficiency disease in Europe in the 1940s and 1950s. It could also have existed for a long time in stable equilibrium with an immune human or primate population and been tipped out of that reservoir by some behavioral change. What is certain is that once having been introduced into vulnerable human populations, AIDS is thriving. Furthermore, the possibility of worldwide spread exists today as never before. The ways in which the AIDS virus is transmitted from host to host resemble the venereal diseases but include many modern features produced by changing sexual mores, transportation and urbanization, and other specific characteristics of this era. Most striking of all are the modern arrangements for transporting infected blood from one person to another, either by the use and abuse of hypodermic needles or in blood transfusion; in this kind of transmission AIDS also mimics another disease, Hepatitis B.

In any discussion of disease propagation, numbers are important, for the ecological strategies of many pathogens involve rapid population growth. Pathogens typically enter the body in small numbers, reproducing there to large numbers and causing sickness. Epidemics are created when pathogens are passed rapidly from host to host, multiplying the numbers of carriers.

In the biological world, the question of the *control* of growth is quite as important as the question of growth itself. Uncontrolled growth of cells in the body is called cancer. Uncontrolled growth of a stable population of bacteria may poison an area of the body where they otherwise live innocuously, and uncontrolled growth of any species in a complex ecosystem may lead to environmental degradation, like overgrazing leading to erosion and the loss of topsoil. Locusts become a scourge when their rate of reproduction suddenly soars. The continuing increase in the number of human beings on this planet is an urgent example of such a danger.

The easiest way to look at uncontrolled growth is in terms of exponential processes and doubling times. All the examples just given can involve exponential growth, but their doubling times vary. Models of exponential growth are stated in terms of powers of two (2^n). If you take two, double it, and double the product repeatedly at some regular time interval, you will find that the numbers rapidly climb terrifyingly high: 2, 4, 8, 16, 32, 64. . . . After ten steps, you have passed the thousand mark. After twenty steps, the million mark. No system can survive very many steps of exponential growth.

The growth of an epidemic becomes visible as incremental growth, the number of fatalities or new cases diagnosed in a given time period. News of 2 or 4 or even 32 new cases does not look very frightening, but the underlying mathematical process becomes recognizable if the same time period that at first yielded 16 or 64 new cases now yields 2,000 or 16,000 or 500,000. If you graph these numbers, a gently rising curve rapidly becomes almost vertical and runs off the paper.

This is what has seemed to be happening with the AIDS epidemic. Official medical awareness of AIDS in the United States is often dated from a published report of five deaths in 1981. By the end of 1987, some 50,000 cases had been reported in the United States, a substantial fraction of the more than 150,000 cases estimated worldwide.

The doubling time for diagnosed cases of AIDS in the United States apparently started at about six months and is now about eighteen months. We do not yet have accurate figures for estimating doubling time in Africa or for specifying different doubling times in different populations. By way of comparison, the doubling time for the common bacterium *E. coli* cultured in the laboratory is twenty to thirty minutes, and for world population it is around forty years. All examples of exponential growth are potentially lethal and likely to end in breakdown. The cancer patient dies; the overpopulated petri dish runs out of medium and is poisoned with wastes; and our planet cannot support the unlimited growth of the human population—perhaps one or two more doubling cycles at best.

With the gradual lengthening of the doubling period, the spread of AIDS is no longer fully exponential. The number of cases is still climbing very fast, but the curve is beginning to steady rather than becoming progressively steeper. This by no means represents a leveling-off, nor does it indicate that the disease is being brought under control or that danger is being reduced. There will only be a true leveling off when, on the average, the number of new cases in a given year equals the level of fatalities—replacement level, Zero AIDS Growth, but still tens and hundreds of thousands of new cases, representing wave after wave of persons infected with the disease. There are still many uncertainties, but the World Health Organization now projects up to three million new cases of AIDS in the next five years. These cases cannot be averted, for most of these individuals are already carrying the virus.

All biological growth processes have the potential for exponential increase, against a very wide range of controls. But exponential processes do not always simply continue to catastrophe. The human embryo doubles in weight within hours and the newborn within months, but the rate of growth declines gradually through adolescence (with a few sudden spurts) and then ceases. How large would a five-year-old be if she continued to grow at the same rate as in the first month after birth? There is a mathematical pattern to this slowing process that can be seen if you graph changes in the doubling period, gradually extending from hours to years. This is the likely pattern of gradual control over AIDS, achieved over a period of years if indeed it can be achieved at all, with a further delay before it would show up in mortality figures. This means that the tragedy and its repercussions in vulnerable communities will continue to take a toll for a long time to come. It also seems likely that the typical doubling time is necessarily different in different kinds of communities, so that a slight slowing in growth rate corresponds to greater coverage, like the flow of a river that moves swiftly in a gully and more slowly as it spreads out onto a broad floodplain. A more abrupt cutoff to the graph could be achieved only by the kind of technical breakthrough that scientists now warn us not to hope for.

Species vary in their reproductive strategies. Human population has been rising slowly and steadily since the beginning of the Common Era, but the reason it is increasing so rapidly now is that our species was able to survive with a much higher death rate than we have today. Reduce deaths, and births begin to look cancerous. In general, the larger species (whales, bears, humans) maintain population balances with relatively few offspring, many of which survive, while smaller species often produce vast numbers of offspring very quickly, most of which die off. The many offspring/many deaths strategy seems wasteful, but it allows for quick evolution.

Thus it is that a small number of cases of some new disease must command immediate attention. If this disease is biologically transmitted, it may spread incredibly rapidly. The ultimate death rate for a disease will depend on (1) the life cycle and rate of increase of the pathogen, (2) the mechanism whereby the pathogen moves from host to host and the speed and frequency of this mechanism, and (3) the effect of the pathogen on the body and the defenses the body is able to erect. Causes of death that are not biologically transmitted are much less worrying because they are not likely to be backed up by the mathematics of growth: death in earthquakes is not catching.

It is absolutely certain that an exponential increase in AIDS fatalities or even infections could not proceed indefinitely, and cannot indeed increase to the logical limit of extinction. Behavioral differences within the species mean that the niche in which the disease is expanding is not uniform, and it is already changing. Even bubonic plague ceased its exponential spread after killing more than a quarter of the population of Europe. But the exponential spread of a disease can proceed to the point of disabling a nation or an economic system. It is already certain that AIDS will cause hundreds of thousands of deaths, even while its doubling time is being slowly extended. Waiting for the epidemic to establish a natural equilibrium was the only response available in the Middle Ages to epidemic diseases, but today too many other equilibria are threatened. Today too we have the possibility of deliberately changing the population dynamics of the pathogen by altering its environment—most immediately, the external environment, in which human behavior determines its transmission from host to host. At the same time, medical research is gradually moving toward ways of altering by medication the internal environment of the human body where the virus multiplies and destroys.

3

THE HUMAN

IMMUNE SYSTEM

■

THE BODY, a community of some seventy-odd trillion cells, is like a miniature ecosystem. Within its boundaries, many types of cells coexist, each with a wide range of interrelated and interdependent activities that must be maintained in balance. In the nineteenth century Claude Bernard, the founder of modern physiology, pointed out that the body devotes many of its resources to the rather conservative goal of maintaining a constant internal environment, in spite of a ceaseless turnover of materials passing through and the repair, production, and death of cells. The sense of self is indirectly related to this continuity, an identity of pattern and information bridging a steady turnover of substance.

It is the maintenance of constancy, dubbed *homeostasis* by the American physiologist Walter Cannon, that is the *raison d'être* of many of the body's physiological systems. For example, the respiratory system is responsible for maintaining an appropriate balance in the body's oxygen account, which is constantly being drawn on to meet the metabolic expenditures of organs and tissues. Homeostasis requires an input of energy to do the work of maintaining constancy, and of materials to sustain and repair the structure of the living machine. These needs are satisfied by the digestive system's orderly tangle of pipes and pouches, an elaborate refinery and nutrient mill which takes the crude ore of food and extracts energy and useful chemical building blocks. A predictable consequence of all this metabolic and digestive activity is the generation of by-products, some of which are potentially toxic. The excretory organs, after a thrifty recycling of what can be kept and reused, identify and sewer wastes. The requirements for the timely pickup and delivery of nutrients, wastes, hormones, and a host of other chemical signals are served in each person by the circulatory system's miles of tubing and the changing rhythms of its central pump, the heart. A continuous and largely unconscious monitoring, analysis, and coordination of temperature, hormonal levels, blood sugar, appetites, and heartbeat is indispensable to the body's self-maintenance. Much of this is regulated by the nervous system, a network of input/output terminals, cables, and biocalculators presided over by the brain, a sophisticated and powerful biocomputer.

All of the diverse mechanisms that are marshaled for the maintenance of homeostasis are based on one central regulatory principle: negative feedback. Simply put, negative feedback provides for self-correction, so that if a system undergoes a change in one direction—a drop in temperature, for example—control mechanisms are activated that produce a change in the opposite direction. Any homeostatic system has a set point about which the controlled parameter fluctuates. When the system deviates from the set point by more than a certain amount, a sensor detects the change or its consequences and initiates corrective action.

In addition to sophisticated physiological processes, the very architectural plan of the body is also important for maintaining a constant internal environment. The body, like a fortress, is designed to keep things out, but instead of walls, moats, and turrets, the body's barrier is its exterior epithelium, whose various manifestations clothe all of its surfaces. Everyone is aware of the tough, relatively thick skin that covers the head, trunk, and extremities. But there are also the sleek, delicate mucous membranes which, while more vulnerable than skin, wrap and unequivocally separate the body's "inner outer" spaces from its true interior. Paradoxical as it may seem, air inflating the lungs, water transiting the esophagus, food digesting in the intestine, semen entering the vagina, and fecal matter passing through the rectum are all "outside the body." This is fortunate. Prolonged exposure of unprotected inner tissues to something as seemingly innocuous as water would cause their cells to bloat and burst, and naked tissues would be damaged by direct exposure to air with its high concentrations of reactive oxygen. Similarly, it is essential that the lining of the alimentary canal keep the processes of digestion safely confined "outside" the body. Otherwise, the versatile and potent mixture of digestive enzymes necessary to break down foodstuffs would damage delicate and vulnerable inner tissues.

The protective epithelium is also the first line of defense against a different but equally grave threat to the integrity of the body. Each of us is like a planet carrying its own small ecosystem on its surface, separated from the core. We all host a large and dynamic microbial community. Bacteria can be found busily coating our teeth with plaque, lurking in competitive company with other tiny creatures in the lungs, and living by the billions in our guts, many of them performing useful services. At each of these sites, there is a fierce struggle to carve out and hold a resource niche, but as long as the skin holds, most of these battles are intermicrobial, fought outside the body, and benign. Only a relative handful of the vast range of microbes are able to cause mischief from outside, attaching themselves to the skin or mucous membranes or even burrowing their way through.

When, however, the exterior epithelium is breached or compromised by whatever means, the inner space of the body becomes available for colonization. To the intensely opportunistic, competition-driven microbial community, the interior of the body represents an El Dorado of resources for growth and reproduction. Since the number and variety of organisms capable of exploiting access to this rich lode of inner resources can be great, infection of the interior is a likely outcome of any breach. Clearly, the introduction and growth of a new and different population of life forms in the delicately balanced milieu of the body represents a significant change and has the potential for causing serious imbalances. The immune system is responsible for combating threats to homeostasis and the maintenance of self posed by the invasion of life forms that are nonself. It plays the decisive role in determining whether an infection will flourish and cause disease or fail to prosper and dwindle.

While some systems of the body, such as the circulatory system, have been well understood for a long time, scientists are still discovering new subtleties in the immune system, a complex and interacting network of many cell types whose function is to guard the body against colonization by foreign organisms. Its success can be traced first to the extraordinary precision with which it can distinguish between self and nonself, and second, to its capacity to tailor its defenses to counter an extraordinarily diverse range of specific threats. What we see here is the relationship between a complex and long-lived organism and the multitudes of much simpler organisms whose generations are so short and their numbers so large that they evolve very rapidly. The counter-strategy to these constantly varying and highly specific threats is flexibility, the capacity to benefit from experience—to adapt within a lifetime as well as across generations—that characterizes not only the human brain but also the human immune system.

The intrusion of an alien presence—a pathogen, which may be as small as a virus or as large as a protozoan— into the familiar landscape of the self triggers a rapid and usually effective immune response that consists of three phases: recognition, amplification, and attack. Diversity is the basis of the flexible response needed to meet the challenge of the constantly evolving variety of pathogens. The developmental process that results in the formation of an immune system does not produce a homogeneous and unvarying population of cells. Instead, a maximum amount of diversity is created by an extraordinary process of genetic rearrangement. Just as the troops of an army are organized into discrete, distinctive, and recognizable units such as squads and platoons, the body produces tens of billions of specialized immune cells in a myriad of functional units called clones. All members of a particular clone arise from the same cell and are identical to one another. They differ from members of other clones in subtle but significant ways about which more will be said shortly. Any one of the body's standing repertoire of hundreds of thousands of clones may contain as few as one or as many as several thousand member cells.

The example of what happens when the immune system swings into action to combat an infection by one of those virulent new strains of flu that appear every ten or twenty years, when our bodies have learned to resist the previous model, provides a good framework for understanding its normal operation. Viruses have the common characteristic of being very small and lacking the machinery to reproduce themselves. They must find suitable host cells, recognizing them by specific molecules on their exterior surface, enter them, and redirect their metabolism to the support of viral reproduction. Since medical science can do little against virus infections except alleviate discomfort, recovery depends on the immune system, particularly on the teamwork of three types of cells—the specialized clones of T cells, the antibody-producing B cells, and the generalist macrophages—that play different and key roles in mounting an immune response. Within the broad category of T cells (cells produced in the thymus gland), there is a further division of labor, with a number of important subcategories such as helper T cells, which are essential for the initiation and amplification of immune responses; cytotoxic (or killer) T cells, which can kill cells bearing foreign antigens; and suppressor T cells, which can turn off or decrease immune responses when the threat is past.

The recognition phase of the immune response is prefaced by encounters between pathogens and macrophages. The macrophage surface is the Krazy Glue of the immune system: most things—viruses, bacteria, and other cells—will stick to it. Since there are tens of billions of macrophages and macrophage-like cells distributed all through the body's tissues, it is inevitable that free-floating influenza virus as well as cells infected with flu will encounter and adhere to such cells.

Cells interact by touch, you might even say by embrace. Both immune cells and invading cells circulate in search of the appropriate significant other to bond to—and, like some human beings in such a search, they respond primarily to externals, recognizing outward clues that identify their target. The clues are molecules on the cell surface, called *antigens*, whose shapes are highly specific. Unlike the Krazy Glue macrophages, specialized immune cells have specialized receptors on their surfaces. All of the receptors on a given cell (and all other members of the same clone) are identical and will fit only particular antigens. Specific immune cells recognize pathogens by the presence of specific antigens on their surface.

Thus, while any of the body's non-specific macrophages can bond to particles of a new flu virus, only the members of a particular clone of T or B cells can do so. This means that individual T and B cells are extremely finicky. The relationship between receptors and the antigens they bind is analogous to the relationship between locks and keys. Just as a given lock will accept only a key with a very particular shape, the receptors on a particular B cell or T cell will bind only to an antigen whose shape precisely fits into the receptor. In fact, different subcategories of T cells, each in its own way, take this sort of fastidiousness a step further. The T cell's receptor can recognize and bind to its antigen only when the antigen is associated with a host cell such as a macrophage, or possibly another cell in which the virus is hidden. To a T-cell receptor, an antigen in isolation is an incomplete key which becomes whole only when it is associated with a characteristic type of molecule present on the surface of a host cell. It is a striking paradox of the immune system that its T-cell arm can only recognize the strange in the context of the familiar.

The association of flu or any foreign antigen with molecules of the macrophage surface completes the structure of an antigen key that can enter a lock-and-key association with any helper T cells that have matching receptors. Such T cells link up with macrophages through these antigen bridges. This initiates a molecular conversation in the immune system which can have lethal consequences for flu, the intruding pathogen. The detection of the pathogen during the recognition phase by members of an appropriate clone results in the production during the amplification phase of the specific forces needed to counter the invading pathogen.

These prefatory stages culminate in the attack phase, in which antibody molecules course through the body seeking out and locking onto the virus—which they recognize by means of the antigens on its surface, rather as a uniform makes it possible to recognize soldiers of an enemy army without detailed examination—and destroying it or preventing it from bonding with host cells. This is an important factor in eliminating the pathogen from the host. Even in the case of viruses that have already lodged within the body's own cells and subverted their normal functions, turning them into virus factories, tiny flags of antigen remain on the cell surface marking them for destruction by the system's own highly targeted killer T cells.

A great many processes are going on at the same time, as different kinds of cells and specialized molecules are produced to play their different but interdependent roles. Understanding these processes is important both in get-ting a picture of the complex coordination involved and also because each step or process suggests a possible point of intervention. The encounter that involves T cell, antigen, and macrophage stimulates the macrophage to produce interleukin I, a protein factor that makes it possible for helper T cells to make interleukin II. This key hormone of the immune system promotes the multiplication of activated T cells, both helpers that support even further production and killers whose receptors bind to flu. Helper T cells also send out a veritable cornucopia of protein factors that orchestrate the immune response, such as gamma interferon, which can improve the ability of macrophages to display antigen in ways that T cells recognize and which, incidentally, makes all kinds of cells less good factories for virus production. Other factors are obligatory signals that must be present in order for those B cells whose receptors match up with flu virus components to multiply and become antibody-producing "factory" cells called plasma cells, each of which can make and ship out on the order of a million antibody molecules a minute. These antibodies bind to particles of influenza virus, marking them and blocking their ability to attach themselves to cells of the host and reproduce, so that instead they wait to be engulfed by a macrophage or some other member of an ever-lurking force of white blood cells specialized to digest antibody-labeled pathogens.

When the patient recovers from flu, the infection is first blocked and then eliminated from the bloodstream, but in the process the few viral particles initially picked up in casual contact have been multiplied into uncounted millions. The human host, who has been quite uncomfortable for days or weeks, has almost certainly spread the virus further. Indeed, every few decades a strain of influenza virus develops into an epidemic that produces thousands of casualties. From the point of view of the individual human patient, the immune system has defeated the virus. But if the virus has spread further, the interlude of a few viral generations in a particular host was a success from the standpoint of the virus.

This particular host will not suffer from this strain of virus again, however, for the immune system is endowed with "memory," that enables it to store information about encounters with specific pathogens. Immunologic memory can be thought of as a kind of learning, whereby the body learns to anticipate likely dangers which can increase the speed and intensity of subsequent responses. Although quite different from the kind of memory used by the brain to store a telephone number or recall a name, it is the basis for acquired immunities, including those artificially produced by vaccination. The multiplication of B cells, mediated by helper T cells which have bound flu-associated antigens, produces an important additional benefit which is the basis of memory. Some of the B cells do not become antibody-secreting plasma cells, but are stockpiled as "memory" B cells against the possibility that the same type of influenza virus will be encountered at some future date. Such stockpiling means that a future flu infection will meet a much larger initial pool of B cells that can recognize it, reproduce themselves, and make antibodies specifically able to combat the virus, so the virus would have to try to establish an infection in the face of a massive and rapidly mobilized population of anti-flu memory B cells. The stockpiling phenomenon is not limited to B cells. We know that helper and killer T-cell populations specific to flu are also stored against future repeat encounters with the same type of flu virus.

One more facet of the response should be appreciated. The processes of demobilization that follow a campaign may be almost as complex as the mobilization that precedes it. Another group of T cells known as suppressor T cells play an important role in the process. The specificity of the recognition and amplification phases that initiate and expand the immune response is complemented in suppression. Consequently, at the same time the immune system is completing and turning off an immune response to one infection, it can specifically initiate a response to a newly invading, different pathogen.

The immune system performs its multiple tasks constantly and largely invisibly. Only when its initial response is delayed or ineffective are we aware of illness. Only when internal defenses fail do we turn to medical science, and then often only to alleviate discomfort, as from flu, while we wait for the immune system to mobilize. Like any homeostatic system, the immune system goes into action to correct an undesirable internal change and to return the system to the normal state, but unlike most homeostatic systems the immune system has the capacity to adjust its state of readiness to make its reaction faster.

The keys to the effective operation of the cooperative community of interdependent elements that comprise the immune system are recognition, regulation, and communication. Medical textbooks document the costs of operational failures in this network of interactions. Various forms of payment discharge the due bill; they include increased susceptibility to infection, cancers, allergies, and autoimmune diseases such as lupus, where the system has trouble distinguishing self from nonself. A number of important diseases, such as diabetes and arthritis, are also believed to be substantially autoimmune. In most of these examples the malfunction is difficult to pinpoint. However, given the importance and interdependence of control elements in orchestrating an immune response, one can readily appreciate that the defensive capacity of the whole system could be effectively neutralized by removal of a pivotal regulatory element.

4

THE NICHE

OF AIDS

■

THE NICHE in which the AIDS virus is spreading with such dramatic speed does not include any organisms, like snails or fleas, other than human beings, nor does it include spaces like air-conditioning systems or pools, where it could live and reproduce independently. With a few exceptions, it lives all of its life cycle within the human body and depends on interactions between human beings to travel from host to host, from bloodstream to bloodstream. Thus, its niche is heavily dependent on behavior and custom. Because human cultural development has linked the entire population of this planet in a single intercommunicating system, AIDS has the potential for transmission throughout that entire system. All of the documented modes of transmission of AIDS, except through the placenta, are based on voluntary behavior, shaped by learning and influenced by culture. The most common form of transmission of the AIDS virus is through sexual intimacy, with the multiple use of intravenous needles and syringes increasing in importance.

The niche in which AIDS is transmitted depends on the occurrence of certain acts within this huge interlocking net of interactions, and is affected by any factor that changes events of transmission, ranging from the cost of air travel to the use of condoms, and including the vast diversity of attitudes and practices concerning sex, medical care, and the use of drugs. Sexual intimacy and needle sharing differ in many ways, but both involve learning and therefore the texture of the network of transmission is by no means uniform, as different biological possibilities are expressed in different cultural contexts.

Although we share much of the mechanics of reproduction with other species, our sexuality is not particularly animal-like but rather is distinctively human, contrasting in important ways with the mechanisms of fertilization in other species. If you compare human sexuality to that of most other mammals (we can leave the birds and bees out of this discussion), you immediately encounter a major contrast: most mammalian sexuality is locked into the estrus cycle, whereby the female is receptive to copulation only during brief periods of high fertility which are indicated to the male by odor or other cues. It is characteristic of human beings that sex is no longer directly attached to reproduction. Instead, sexuality has evolved to have a potential for enjoyment regardless of fertility, and the pleasure associated with sex underlies other kinds of intimacy and attachment.

Setting sex free from the fertility cycle may have been very important in human evolution, strengthening the bonds between males and females to allow the development of the protective family as childhood dependency became longer. The original separation of sexuality and fertility happened far back in human evolution, so the invention of modern contraception can be seen as the logical development of a process long under way: sex as intimacy, pleasure, and release of tension, as a characteristically human development. This is part of the emergence of humanness, the shift from highly specific and programmed behaviors to much more general ones that can be reshaped in dozens of different ways.

Since Freud, we can see the sources of adult sexuality

in very early infant behavior: the infant sucking passion-
ately at breast or thumb; the toddler learning the satisfactions of controlling elimination, holding on and letting go, fullness and release; the nursery schooler avidly
exploring genitals and wondering who has what. The
pleasures of touching and being touched also start in
infancy, and it is possible to recognize a sexual compo-
nent in all sensory satisfactions: stroking a cat, swaying
to rhythmic music, tasting a delicious meal. As a result,
all of the senses—sight, sound, smell, and taste, as well
as touch—play a role in sexual arousal and response.
Similarly, all of the body's surfaces and orifices, particularly the mouth and the anus, have roles along with
the genitals in giving and receiving pleasure. Limiting
eroticism to unadorned vaginal intercourse, because it is
the only expression of sexuality leading directly to reproduction, narrows the human potential drastically and,
particularly for women, may exclude real fulfillment.

Sexual behavior is extremely variable from person to
person and from culture to culture, but there are some
continuities to be discovered behind the diversity. These
are essential keys to understanding how human sexuality
provides a niche for disease and how human sexuality
can be altered. All human cultures seem to work from
clues offered by biology, but then they go on to select
and elaborate. There is no human culture, even where
body covering is not needed for warmth, that does not
ornament the human body in some way, whether with
fabric or paint or scarification. Similarly, there is no
culture that lacks a concept of modesty about some body
parts or functions, though the choices contrast a great
deal. When outsiders first arrived in many areas of New
Guinea, native women seemed to them naked and therefore shameless, because they did not realize that the net
bags the women wore draped across their backs were
serving the purposes of decorum. In Bali, urination was
traditionally not a matter for concealment, but eating
solid food in public was highly embarrassing. The Old
Testament suggests that a man's head uncovered before

God is like an uncircumcised penis. Americans traveling in Iran often scandalized their hosts by the indecency of blowing their noses audibly in public.

Cultures also vary greatly in when and where and with whom they permit the expression of sexuality, but there are always some prohibitions. A man may be forbidden to sleep with his sister but allowed to have sex with virtually anyone else, or he may be forbidden even to look at most of the females in the community. He may be instructed, as an important part of his initiation into manhood, to have sex with young boys—or he may be risking his life if he does so.

This diversity might suggest that since no particular rule is fully shared by all human beings and humans seem to succeed in living together and reproducing with an incredible variety of rules, perhaps all rules should be discarded, or perhaps only a minimal form of the incest taboo (which does occur almost everywhere) should be retained. But this conclusion misses the essential common element of selection and elaboration: The rules may vary but there are always rules, rules that have to be learned by each child born into the society. *The expression of human sexuality is never just natural*. It is always shaped in some way.

Another cross-cultural similarity that is important is the metaphorical relationship that often exists between sex and other kinds of behavior. It is almost impossible to deal with one behavioral domain in isolation from others and from other cultural styles and values. Human beings use sex to express their feelings, feelings of anger as well as tenderness. Eroticism can express a cultural value placed on risk or on achievement, can convey defiance or comfort, can be an assertion of identity or an expression of dominance—and the same kinds of issues arise in relation to drug use. If in one culture, sex or drugs is linked to courage and risk taking, the risk of death from AIDS may be seen as an additional challenge to manhood; and if the defiance of authority is a key motivation behind sex or drug use, authoritative advice on precautions will not be accepted. If self-sacrifice is romanticized, the risk of disease may be embraced as an alternative route to self-sacrifice.

In recent years we have been changing the rules and meanings associated with sex. Superficially it looks as if all the changes involve a loosening of repression. As a society we have become much more tolerant of sex outside marriage or before marriage and of homosexuality and masturbation, and we read books that suggest new and exotic positions and recommend oral sex. But we have also accepted new sets of limits and expectations: a woman may wear the tiniest of bikinis but she must "cover up" the natural odors of her body; a man may bulge in the crotch but agonize to conceal a bulge a few inches higher up. We have stronger prohibitions on coercive sex than ever before—in many states, although a man may sleep with someone he is not married to, he may not insist on sex with his wife if she declines. We are making real efforts to prevent rape and child molestation, instead of simply covering up areas of sexual violence that must have been routine in the past. And we expect individuals to be sexually active and skilled: college girls worry if they are still virgins at twenty, men worry about losing their potency, and men are increasingly expected to be concerned for the sexual satisfaction of female partners. People used to worry about "impure thoughts," but now they worry about insufficient ingenuity.

Nature does not just take its course. It cannot be a simple shift to permissiveness that decrees that in America today, sexual acts that would have been condoned (by collusive concealment) twenty years ago can destroy political candidates. Teenagers may be newly sexually active, but they still have clear ideas about what kinds of behavior fit their own standards.

In other words, although the "sexual revolution" does involve a wider range of sexual activity, with greater possibilities for disease transmission, it does not represent a replacement of regulated by unregulated sexuality.

The rules have been changing and they can change again. The invention of new limitations and elaborations is what has made our sexual behavior human. It is important to see sexual expression as variable in many different ways, not as varying on a single dimension between permissiveness and repression. It is similarly essential to understand that even illegal activities like drug use or prostitution are not without rules, for every human group surrounds activities important to it with customs and expectations.

You don't need a great many explicit rules to establish a principle of lawfulness that permits a workable human environment. It is entirely possible to shape biological sexuality into a vast range of pleasurable elaborations, and also to limit it to protect the weak from exploitation and to control the transmission of disease. Possible, but by no means automatic; easier across generations than within a single generation whose habits are already shaped.

There are interesting analogies to be found in the ways in which different cultures deal with stimulants and drugs, for the desire to alter mental states by the use of substances from mescaline to coffee and from nicotine to heroin is another recurrent theme of human elaboration on biology. Each of these presents real dangers to health, but within the human range it is clear that some American prejudices and preferences are rather arbitrary, that substance use is less likely to turn to abuse when hedged about by ceremony and courtesy, and that prohibition brings its own set of dangers and promotes the values of defiance. In other words, it should be possible to adjust the social patterns of drug use to reduce the real dangers presented by these different kinds of drugs, including the economic exploitation by dealers. A puritanical condemnation of drug use as a search for pleasure is not the best place to start.

Ironically, the particular attitudes toward sex that have historically characterized Western culture now represent a handicap in understanding the human characteristics of sexuality. Christianity has been more negative and secretive about sex than virtually any other tradition, for while all high cultures limit sexuality and elaborate on some forms of asceticism and self-control, Christianity has in many periods suggested that all sexual activity and all erotic pleasure are deplorable. Islamic cultures, which seem extreme to Westerners in the limitations they put even on the imagination of possible partners, are still entirely clear that sex is to be enjoyed.

Americans entered the twentieth century largely as a band of sexual illiterates, like a tribe whose experience of music is limited to a six-toned whistle and a drum. We are still liable to lapse into repression—or reactions to repression—and to be haunted by the imagination of sex as a shapeless and uncontrollable force, hidden by darkness but knocking down all restraints in its way. There have been times when the speculative intellect was treated in much the same manner.

By a coincidence of timing, the early spread of the AIDS epidemic was associated in the United States with homosexuality, to a degree that became one more line of defense against realistic discussion, since there are still those who believe that AIDS is a "gay plague." Gay sex needs to be seen in the context of human sexual diversity and elaboration, rather than set off as a separate phenomenon.

Of all aspects of sexuality, homosexual eroticism has been, since the era when it was important in ancient Greece, among the most heavily repressed in Western culture and often subject to savage penalties. There have always been men and women, however, many of them married, who found physical and psychological intimacy with members of the same sex, and there have always been social contexts in which such preferences were protected or valued. The tolerance for sexual elaboration that has tended to follow centers of playfulness and inquiry has often included homosexuality, but on the whole public denial persisted until the middle of this century.

In the United States, the focal incident in the change of attitude toward homosexuality was a police raid in 1969 on a gay bar in New York's Greenwich Village, called the Stonewall Inn. The raid began in the old pattern: a neighborhood with a tradition of nonconformity; a group of largely closeted homosexuals whose behavior was so defined as to make them permanently vulnerable; and a group of police who knew where to find them whenever they wanted engaged in a periodic bout of persecution, like Cossacks occasionally turning to a pogrom. Laws forbidding particular forms of sexual behavior don't work well, they tend to settle to long-term oscillations between tolerated but concealed violation on the one hand and repression on the other. But this raid turned into a riot that changed the definitions and triggered the process called gay liberation. The gay affirmation of rights and the search for subcultural definition that followed were hardly a decade old when the first cases of AIDS were observed, but an earlier case, now recognized in retrospect, was actually recorded in 1969, before the gay liberation movement was under way.

There is no necessary association between AIDS and homosexuality, and the AIDS epidemic could have been spread around America and Europe, as it was in central Africa and as it continues to spread slowly and steadily, primarily by heterosexual contacts. However, gay liberation represented a significant cultural change and we are still learning to understand it.

There is still a great deal that is unknown about the forms that gay sex might take in a society where it was not proscribed, since virtually the entire gay community grew up with guilt and self-rejection and secrecy, and the reactions to these have been factors in emerging sexual styles. Some characteristics, however, can be predicted for male-male sexuality for a long time to come. It appears that females are more concerned on the average with sex as an aspect of sustained and caring relationships, while males are on the average more interested in the pleasures of transient encounters. Given an evolutionary pattern in which females with children became increasingly dependent on the presence of the father, this makes good evolutionary sense.

Whether or not these tendencies are biologically given, our cultural expectation is that the woman will look for stable monogamy and the man for freedom. The traditional family for which conservatives pine has long moderated its monogamy by the double standard. In situations where male preferences govern, the number of transient encounters does seem to increase, including the wholesale rape that often occurs in warfare. Among homosexuals, lesbians tend to confirm this pattern by forming long-term partnerships which are especially striking in the absence of most of the social pressures that sustain marriage. On the other hand, while many gay men do form long-term partnerships, it sometimes seemed as if 1970s-style gay sex was an enactment of a male fantasy common to heterosexuals as well, regardless of preference or partner: uncommitted, impersonal, profligate sex. Another way of looking at this is to notice that heterosexual sex, if it is to be satisfying to both partners, always involves a degree of compromise between different tempos and rhythms, a certain lack of comprehension of the other's body which has to be bridged; this kind of compromise sets constraints of a kind that may be reduced for gays.

Thus, it seems probable, looking at the cross-cultural evidence, that gay sex as it developed in the 1970s represented an intensive exploration of only some of the possible dimensions of gay sexuality. Styles of male-male sexuality at different times and places have varied a good deal. In some cultures, from classical Greece to the New Guinea highlands, most individuals are expected to be somewhat bisexual, while in others, sex between males is heavily prohibited so that only those with very strong homosexual preferences ever act on them. In effect, our particular way of classifying sexual preferences is an artifact of cultural expectations. It has been quite common to associate different sexual preferences with different stages of the life cycle, allowing for serial bisexuality. In other places, homosexuality takes its place within the same two-track system of sexuality that recurs in heterosexual relations in many societies—a home track of stable sex for respectability, mutual support, and reproduction; a fast track for romance or escape.

At different times and places the practices of homosexuals, like those of heterosexuals, have also differed, sometimes emphasizing manual or oral stimulation rather than anal intercourse, and heterosexual practices and competences have varied in the same kinds of ways. There is also variation on whether given individuals regularly take the active or passive role or whether there is alternation. All of the forms of stimulation used by gay men with each other are sometimes used by heterosexual couples, but because of the location of the prostate gland, to be penetrated anally provides an extremely intense stimulation for males, leading to practices such as fisting, the insertion of a full fist into the rectum. The anus is an erogenous zone for both males and females, but anal intercourse is apparently commonest in heterosexual couples as a preference of bisexual men who are accustomed to penetrating anally, or as a way of avoiding conception.

Looking at male homosexuality cross-culturally does suggest a predictably lower emphasis on permanent pairing, but it also makes clear that the sexual style of gay communities in the 1970s and early 1980s was a specific historic phenomenon that might not have endured in a society tolerant of homosexual preferences over time. The lid was taken off, that which had been forbidden was permitted, and the explosion lasted for a decade. Some gay men became sexual athletes, and group sex with multiple contacts was common, so that we hear of hundreds of different sexual contacts within a year and heterosexual men shake their heads in astonishment. Sex became an expression of unity and solidarity in the gay community, linking hundreds of men to each other, much as it links couples in happy marriages. Gay liberation meant release from loneliness and exclusion, becoming members not of a family but of a movement which rapidly became international.

The styles of gay sex that developed in the 1970s did have a number of characteristics that quite inevitably accelerated the spread of many diseases, including AIDS. A value system and a network of institutions, the bathhouses, emerged that encouraged frequent transient relationships. Multiple contacts and sex with strangers meant that any parasite or disease that entered the pool was likely to be spread to all. Explorations of the anus as an erogenous zone led to a link between mouth and anus—exactly the link that has to be cut to deal with a wide range of intestinal parasites. The lining of the rectum is more fragile than the lining of the vagina, so that anal intercourse is far more likely than vaginal intercourse to provide access to the bloodstream of the receptive partner, whereby AIDS can be transmitted. The escalation of anal intercourse by fisting increases the danger.

One way of thinking of the historic role of the gay community in the early spread of the epidemic in America and Europe is to compare a frontier community, where homesteads are many hours apart so that visiting takes place rarely, to a densely populated town. A rumor that would fly through the town in a day might take a year to percolate through the more diffuse community. The townspeople would tend to accept the rumor more readily, because each one would hear it from multiple sources. But gradually the rumor would be passed through the frontier community as well. Similarly, children in nursery schools and their parents may be the first to pick up a new strain of cold or flu, but although the infection spreads more gradually among adults outside, spread it does. There have been important variations in texture in the network of interactions that makes the transmissions of AIDS possible, a network of which we are all a part. Gay bathhouses became focal points of infection. More recent focal points are the "shooting galleries" in which many addicts use the same needles. When blood products are not tested, blood banks can play a similar role, as can centers of prostitution. These focal points have functioned to amplify the epidemic, accelerating the process of spread and creating multitudes of carriers who can pass the disease on, in a second wave of transmissions, often in different settings or by different kinds of behavior.

From the first appearance of AIDS in Africa and in African patients in Europe, it has been a heterosexual disease. It now seems clear that AIDS will spread among heterosexuals somewhat more slowly than it did among homosexuals, but equally inexorably. The access of semen to the bloodstream is less predictable in vaginal sex, but clearly some virus particles do insinuate themselves through the mucous membranes of the genitalia, probably through tiny, invisible lesions. This occurs much more easily when there are already lesions or inflammations of the mucous membranes. In fact, all of the other sexually transmitted diseases should be regarded as increasing vulnerability to AIDS. In the United States so far, the disease appears to move more easily from males to females than vice versa, with relatively few female-to-male transmissions and very few female-to-female transmissions. One common pattern is that a man contracts AIDS from a drug connection and passes it on sexually to his wife, who transmits it through the placenta to an unborn child. In societies that are organized so that men depend on prostitutes, they may function as analogues to the bathhouses in gay sex, the place where all the trails of infection cross, perhaps because of the co-occurrence of other infections. In warfare or in situations of rapid urbanization when men earn cash income by migratory labor and women remain at home in their villages planting food crops, it may take only a very small population of infected prostitutes in the capital to spread disease through the hinterlands or across national boundaries.

Because the AIDS virus moves through the body in the blood, the most direct way to contract the disease is by introducing the virus particles themselves in quantity directly into the bloodstream, where they then seek the right kinds of cells to take refuge in and use as a base for reproduction. Blood-to-blood transmission might possibly occur in accidents or in the context of traditional ways of treating the body, like circumcision or tattooing, but it is very much assisted by modern practices that involve direct access to the bloodstream in transfusions or in intravenous injections of medication. The same modern technology that allows the use of the bloodstream to diffuse a medication rapidly through the body also allows the intensification of drug use: instead of taking drugs in through ingestion or through the mucous membranes by inhalation, drugs can be shot directly into the veins.

In the United States AIDS is no longer transmitted to a significant degree through medical transfusions or blood products, but for a period of about five years it was, and each individual infected by medical treatment has been a potential bridgehead of the disease into the population at large, a random sowing of the virus through the nation that cut across race and class, ethnicity and sexual preference. When disease is transmitted by medical practice, it is called *iatrogenic*, disease caused by the physician, occasionally by neglect but in this case through lack of knowledge. The iatrogenic spread of AIDS in blood products made it an equal opportunity disease and helped drive home an awareness of the range of danger and of the fact that it was unconnected to moral responsibility. Newspapers reported the death from AIDS of a nun who had had a transfusion; hemophiliacs, including children, developed the disease; and people remembered that the President of the United States had had multiple transfusions in 1981. Iatrogenic AIDS continues in parts of the world where the efficacy of a medication is trusted only when it is injected into a vein—the modern form of magic—often by an untrained folk practitioner with limited equipment. In third world countries, including most of Africa, there are usually no funds to test blood for the presence of the virus, but transfusions are sometimes the only way a life can be saved. Thus, transfusion AIDS remains a danger in many countries.

In the United States today, the overwhelmingly most important form of nonsexual transmission is among drug users who share needles. The sharing of needles is partly an artifact of attempts to control drug use, since possession of a syringe, like possession of heroin itself, is grounds for arrest in many places. This leads addicts to shoot up immediately after purchase, using and reusing rented "works" in shooting galleries, but there are other factors: the inconvenience of carrying fragile syringes, the suspicions of dealers who want to be sure that a purchaser is really a user, the companionship involved in shooting up together. Ironically, sharing needles, perhaps with one other person rather than in a shooting gallery, is common among occasional users who do not think of themselves as addicts. Intravenous drug use is a difficult behavior to change because it is supported by chemical addiction, but needle sharing is a more pliable behavior and there are already experiments under way to supply clean needles and syringes and to remove the laws that create the environment for needle sharing. An alternative approach is teaching addicts to clean their "works" with solutions of household bleach.

As with the gay community, the significance of the spread of AIDS among addicts was masked by the stigmatization of the group at risk. Similarly, there was relatively little concern about heroin addiction in American society until it began to spread to middle-class teenagers. In other words, the attitudes that permitted the neglect of the AIDS epidemic in the first few crucial years are a repeat of the self-righteous indifference of the past. We are still, as a society, so preoccupied with moral disapproval of drugs that it blocks our capacity to address the problem, yet drug abuse is itself life-threatening. Heroin addiction, even though it is also seen as a threat to white society, has continued to be closely related to poverty and discrimination, the factors that lock minority youths out of other lifestyles and ambitions. Addiction defines individuals as criminal, leading to a variety of forms of violence and prostitution, and putting users outside the range of public health education—it's not easy for officials to give credible advice to individuals locked into a behavior that is defined as criminal. AIDS is transmitted by the needles used and shared by addicts and is amplified by the other medical and socioeconomic problems of the drug community. Unlike the gay community, the drug culture tends to be highly localized.

Although AIDS has become a global problem, the picture of the niche of AIDS and its transmission outside the body is not a picture of the planet itself but of a network of human interactions that embrace it, only a tiny fraction of all possible interactions. The disease, like the postal and telephone systems, spans the globe, but just as many individuals do not own telephones and never receive mail, so many individuals are only potentially involved in the interactions that transmit AIDS while others are involved in dense and overlapping interchanges. The behaviors that transmit AIDS actually create multiple patterns in different places, so that it is possible to speak of three or four different AIDS epidemics focused in different "risk groups," but together they constitute the niche of AIDS. Like separate oil spills, each is gradually diffused and the boundaries fade in the current, for no risk group is self-contained.

5

THE AIDS
VIRUSES

■

WHEN A PATHOGEN enters the body, it faces the formidable problem of establishing itself before the immune system is sufficiently mobilized to eliminate it. Many pathogens try to outrun immune defenses by multiplying too fast for the immune system to catch up, others change their antigenic clothing, and some even borrow host antigens and masquerade as part of the body. By contrast, Human Immunodeficiency Virus (HIV), the virus family that causes AIDS, tackles the immune system head-on. It actually takes up residence in the immune system and uses its reactions as a vehicle of its own multiplication. HIV infection results in catastrophic loss of the helper T cell population. The decimation of this key regulatory population as a consequence of the body's infection with the AIDS virus produces a collapse of immune defenses, rendering the host easy prey to a number of microbes that would be readily held at bay by a competent immune system.

Clearly the AIDS virus represents the evolution of an extraordinarily successful strategy for evading and subverting host defenses and for exploiting the immune system as its niche within the ecosystem of the body. Once established, the virus makes another smart move. Unlike smallpox or polio, it does not immediately make the host gravely ill. Typically, after a brief episode of relatively mild illness, there is a latent period of seven to ten years which are virtually symptom-free. These apparently healthy carriers continue their normal patterns of life at full vigor, and hence are ideal vectors for spreading the disease. In the few years since recognition of the disease in 1981, it has become apparent that the AIDS epidemic is a plague caused by one of the most insidiously ingenious pathogens in recorded history.

Some years ago, in an interesting and controversial book called *The Selfish Gene*, Richard Dawkins argued that any organism, be it human, insect, or plant, is no more than a disposable machine that genes use to make more genes. Basically, this is a sophisticated restatement of the aphorism that the chicken is just the egg's way of making another egg. In this view Einstein and Picasso are just gene machines. The profound insights of the theory of relativity and the moral majesty of *Guernica* are just a sideshow, incidental to the real work of multiplying, shuffling, and passing on the DNA that created these extraordinary protoplasmic contraptions.

Viruses are the most basic form of gene machines known. A virus is essentially genetic information wrapped up in a protein coat. Although some may have an extra ingredient or two, the basic building plan of all viruses includes nucleic acid, which carries the genetic information, and a protein coat, which forms a protective wrapper around the nucleic acid. The protein coat also acts as an organelle of attachment that enables the virus to bind to an appropriate host cell that can support its reproduction. Viruses are different from other living things in that they do not have the array of complex metabolic machinery necessary for the conduct of the basic processes of life. They can reproduce only by gaining entry into an appropriate type of living cell and exploiting its life processes. Once inside a cell, the virus's library of genetic instructions, carried by its nucleic acid, is used as a blueprint for the fabrication of new virus particles, so the cell is metabolically tricked into becoming a molecular factory for the reproduction of these molecular cuckoos. In the case of many viruses, the reproduction of the virus results in the debilitation and death of the infected cell.

The members of the family of viruses that cause AIDS belong to a category known as *retroviruses*. In addition to HIV, this category contains a number of members that cause cancer in other animals—feline leukemia virus (cats); bovine leukemia virus (cattle); Rous sarcoma virus (chickens)—as well as HTLV-I, that causes a type of T cell leukemia in humans. The retroviruses have invented some variations on the basic pattern of virus reproduction just outlined. The unique feature of retroviruses is the way they transform, store, and subsequently retrieve their genetic information after entering a susceptible host cell. These viruses employ the nucleic acid RNA rather than DNA as their molecular repository of genetic information.

To borrow a familiar phrase, "every schoolboy knows" the following one-way scheme for the flow of genetic information:

$$\circlearrowleft DNA \longrightarrow RNA \longrightarrow Protein$$

This succinct statement, sometimes called the Central Dogma of molecular biology, describes the expression of genetic information in living organisms as diverse as humans, box elders, and bacteria. Decoded, it states that DNA, the genetic information of all living cells, is faithfully copied (replicated) to make more of itself. The expression of the genetic information proceeds by employing the nucleic acid DNA as a template for the precise transcription of RNA, a different type of nucleic acid, which contains precisely the same information as the DNA template. The portion of this RNA known as messenger RNA serves as an intracellular shuttle, taking genetic information to the cell's protein-synthesizing machinery. Messenger RNAs act as the blueprints for the synthesis of an extremely large and diverse ensemble of proteins that are characteristic and distinctive of, and indispensable to, the organism. The form, function, and very nature of the organism is determined by the activities of its proteins. That complement of proteins is the expression of the information in the organism's DNA. Ultimately, it is to differences in the chemical structure of DNA that we can trace the differences between a goose and a gander or a man and a marigold.

Some years ago, the retroviruses forced a revision in the Central Dogma that DNA is the only source of genetic specificity, which strict constructionists would read as, "DNA makes RNA but RNA does not make DNA." Among their protein constituents, retroviruses also include an enzyme called *reverse transcriptase*. This enzyme can use the viral RNA as a template for the synthesis of DNA which has exactly the same genetic information. So retroviruses sing a tune that begins like this: RNA $\longrightarrow$ DNA. This biochemical "transubstantiation" of information will soon be seen to play a critical role in the reproduction of retroviruses.

All of this activity involves biological processes that were unknown until a few years ago. The central role of DNA was discovered in the 1950s, the various kinds of T cells in the immune system began to be understood during the late 1970s, and the first human retrovirus was described by Robert Gallo and his associates in 1978. Most diseases preyed upon human beings for centuries before it was possible to understand them. Although there are indications that this disease has been with us for much longer than we initially thought, epidemic AIDS is a unique case of a problem arising just as powerful technologies and concepts to address it came into being.

The reproductive cycle of a retrovirus, like that of other animal viruses, begins with the virus recognizing and binding to a host cell. The "recognition" is, of course, purely molecular and consists of the virus quite literally bumping into cell surfaces until it encounters a molecular structure on a host cell that snugly fits its receptor. In the case of HIV, the host cell structure sought is CD4, a molecule found on the surface of a number of cell types including helper T cells and macrophage-type cells of the immune system. Once a virus has locked onto the surface of an appropriate cell, the host cell cannot avoid committing what will likely prove a suicidal act: just as Troy took in the horse, the cell internalizes the virus. Once inside, the virus sheds its protein coat and uses its own reverse transcriptase to fashion raw materials appropriated from the host into a DNA copy (a *provirus*) of its RNA. This foreign viral DNA, a molecular "mole" whose role is to lie in wait until the "call" comes, now gets safely incorporated into the well-protected and extensive DNA library of the host cell nucleus. However, this nuclear sanctuary is only relative, for the provirus directs the synthesis of viral proteins, some of which find their way to the exterior surface of the cell where they lodge, tiny molecular tags, distinctively marking the host cell as occupied territory. Thus some infected T cells are eliminated by the immune system itself.

When the time comes to swing into virus production, the provirus will serve as a template for the replication of the virus. Just when that moment comes depends on environmental conditions and varies for different kinds of retroviruses. In the case of HIV-infected helper T cells, the provirus lies in wait until the cell is stimulated from outside to divide. Whereas there are various tricks for doing this in the laboratory, helper T cells are stimulated to divide in the body only when they encounter the antigen for which they are programmed, associated with the surface of a macrophage-type cell. The stimulus to divide switches on the capacity of the HIV provirus to send out genetic instructions that dictate the manufacture of massive numbers of HIV particles. The host cell is converted to a microfactory that promptly and dutifully carries out these instructions. The massive burst of newly synthesized virus particles budding from the cell surface results in the death of the cell. The newly minted HIV particles can infect still other CD4-bearing cells of the host.

HIV does not have to put all of its eggs in the T-helper basket. CD4 molecules decorate the surface of macrophages and many other macrophage-like cells, some of which are part of the central nervous system. Finding receptors on their surfaces, HIV readily infects these cells just as it does helper T cells, once again inhabiting the very cells that should be protecting the body against it. However, even though HIV follows the retrovirus pattern of copying its genes to DNA when it infects macrophages, the pattern of growth is different from that seen in HIV-infected helper T cells. Instead of a latency period followed by an eruption of virus at the time of cell division, with the concomitant death of the host cell, infected macrophages produce a continuous stream of virus particles and are not destroyed in the process.

Some of the virus produced by infected macrophages and triggered by helper T cells spreads the infection within the host by entering additional cells. Any uninfected helper T cell that visits the surface of a virus-producing macrophage for an encounter with antigen will likely be treated to an excellent opportunity to become a host to HIV. Macrophages are migratory cells, recruited to sites of infection by chemical signals, but an infected macrophage invited in by a signaling T cell will bring a burden of unwelcome baggage. Free virus particles in blood and semen, as well as already infected cells, may become agents for the export of the disease to someone else. So again the evolutionary forces that shaped the AIDS virus are seen to capitalize on the biology of the immune system.

The fact that HIV propagates in more than one type of cell, with one rhythm in some types and a different tempo in others, greatly complicates our understanding the dynamics of the infection. Although there are many billions of macrophages and macrophage-like cells susceptible to HIV, the roster is still not complete. Components of the central nervous system are also at risk. In all too many AIDS cases, HIV manages to insinuate itself into the central nervous system, crossing the so-called blood-brain barrier, and infecting CD4-bearing cells there, damaging the brain and producing the AIDS dementias. It is possible that HIV infection of the nervous system paves the way for neurological damage by several different mechanisms. The point here is that the effects, direct and indirect, of HIV-mediated damage to the central nervous system can be predictably catastrophic. It is also apparent that the existence of so many different sites of growth greatly complicates the problem of eliminating a well-entrenched HIV infection from the body.

Simple But Subtle Machines

Because of their lack of basic metabolic machinery, viruses do not enjoy full membership in the club of life. Compared to even the most primitive bacteria, viruses are quite simple. But the simplicity is relative, for any independent entity that has a genetic structure and a capacity for evolution has an impressive absolute complexity and a high information content. So it is with those engines of replication we call viruses. Among the viruses, the biology of HIV is one of the most complex we know. The virus has an outer envelope that is a stripped-down version of the membrane that encases all cells. This outer coat of HIV is a watertight seal studded with many protein molecules that have been shaped by evolution to bind to the CD4 molecule. These are the virus's receptors that allow it to pick out and attach itself to the right kinds of host cell. Within the virus, one finds its genetic information, two molecules of RNA in an inner shell of protein. This genetic redundancy, carrying two complete copies of genetic instructions, is characteristic of retroviruses and extraordinary among viruses. Furthermore, when one examines the organization and content of the information carried by this virus, two striking facts emerge: HIV carries more information than any other known type of retrovirus, and some of this information is devoted to activities of regulation and control that are unique to these viruses.

What emerges from this profile of HIV is an agent that has evolved a number of structural and regulatory features that have fit it to tenant, thus far with devastating success, a new niche. It is essential to learn its characteristics in as short a time as possible, for the more one understands the quirks of its structure and its mode of infection and reproduction, the better the opportunity to design an approach to interdict the transmission and reproduction of the virus.

Since the discovery of HIV in 1983, just two years after AIDS was recognized as a disease, a truly impressive amount of information has been amassed about this new type of retrovirus. The rapidity of the progress can be traced to the extraordinary power of the new techniques of genetic engineering, such as gene cloning and structure determination, and also to newer immunological techniques. These powerful technologies have been applied with dazzling skill by a number of talented investigators. When the history of this epidemic is written, one of the bright spots in what has so far been a dark and dreary pattern of despair will be the performance of the working researchers. Despite the slowness with which administrators made decisions and the early niggardliness of their support, an impressive job has been done.

Where to Find HIVs and Their Relatives

Today we know that there is more than one member of the HIV family, variously distributed on different continents. AIDS caused by the HIV-1 member of the family is the most familiar in Europe, the Americas, and Australia and is most heavily represented in central, east, and, increasingly, southern Africa. HIV-2, a more recently discovered form of the virus, is most heavily concentrated in western Africa. Western Europe, particularly France and the British Isles, has hosted HIV-1–induced AIDS since the 1970s and possibly even earlier. By contrast there are few reported cases in the Soviet Union and the Eastern European block. In the Americas, the United States, Brazil, and the islands of the Caribbean, particularly Haiti, have the highest per capita numbers of AIDS patients. The disease does not yet have major representation in the Pacific basin and the rest of Asia. But the ever-increasing pattern of trade and tourist exchange carries a risk, indeed almost a certainty, that this populous and dynamic area of the world may soon lose its epidemiological immunity, for the spread of the virus precedes the appearance of disease. In fact the disease has already made modest inroads in Australia and in the Philippines.

Another immunodeficiency virus, SIV (Simian Immunodeficiency Virus), distinct from HIV-1 and HIV-2, can be isolated from monkeys indigenous to the African forests. The genetic material of this retrovirus encodes structural and regulatory information that is quite similar to that of the HIVs. The existence of such viruses provides relevant evidence for those who are interested in the origins of AIDS. From a practical point of view, SIV and its simian hosts may also provide a useful animal model for drug and vaccine tests that could not be ethically conducted on human volunteers.

HIV: The Cause of AIDS

What is the factual basis for the conclusion that HIV is the cause of AIDS? Although much more study is necessary in order to say exactly what fraction of HIV-infected individuals will develop AIDS, it is already clear from groups carefully monitored over time that well over 40 percent of those infected with the virus have already progressed to full-blown AIDS. Unfortunately, the rate of conversion to AIDS seems not to decrease with time, but to claim an almost constant fraction of carriers each year. In fact, there is an emerging consensus among epidemiologists that, in the absence of a therapeutic breakthrough, almost all infected people will develop AIDS. While it is true that other viruses can be isolated from some patients, and other patients have bacterial infections such as syphilis, only HIV, with its telltale molecular traces, emerges as the common denominator of all AIDS cases.

Persuasive as such a pattern of association may be, it does not eliminate the possibility that HIV might be present without being the actual cause of disease. However, although it is impossible to experiment directly by deliberately injecting HIV into human beings, there are additional and independent lines of evidence that are convincing.

First, the transfusion of individuals with no risk factors for AIDS with blood or blood products that were later found to contain HIV resulted in infections that tragically progressed to AIDS in hundreds of individuals. This eliminates alternative behavioral causes. Second, in the course of performing experiments, a laboratory worker who was accidentally inoculated with a concentrated preparation of HIV became infected and developed AIDS. Finally, a particularly strong case emerges from studies with monkeys. Infection of monkeys with SIV, which, as we have noted, is very similar to HIV, produces many of the symptoms—swollen lymph nodes, susceptibility to opportunistic infections, a decrease in the number of helper T cells—and the same outcome— death from an AIDS-like disease—seen in HIV-infected AIDS patients.

The SIV experiments are especially convincing because the behavior of experimental animals can be tightly regulated, their history is known, and they are not infected with the host of other viruses and bacteria that some have suspected of being responsible for AIDS in humans. Furthermore, one can use a well-defined stock of SIV to induce simian AIDS. Subsequently, virus can be isolated from afflicted monkeys and shown to cause the same disease when injected into healthy monkeys. All of these findings, the epidemiological and clinical studies of human patients and the model studies in experimental animals, lead one to the inescapable conclusion that HIV infection is the cause of AIDS.

Thinking About an AIDS Vaccine

The technology of vaccination is based on the phenomenon of immunological memory. When the immune system is exposed to a foreign pathogen such as a virus or bacterium, it expands the repertoire of T and B cells that can specifically react against the components of the intruder. However, not all of these cells are expended during the initial encounter; some are stockpiled as a population base of defensive "memory" cells. If at some future time there is reinfection by the same pathogen, it triggers a rapid expansion of this large defensive population and thus confronts a massive and decisive immune response. The virtual elimination of smallpox worldwide and the control of a host of other infectious diseases stand as monuments to the success and versatility of vaccination.

Clearly, one does not vaccinate by injecting healthy people with the infectious form of a pathogenic microbe. The trick of making a good vaccine lies in the ability to present the body with a form of the microbe that is recognizable to the immune system but unable to cause disease. There are four approaches to this problem. The oldest of these involves inoculation with an organism that is immunologically closely related to the pathogen, but does not cause disease in the host. The efficacy of this approach was first demonstrated almost two hundred years ago by the English physician Edward Jenner, who showed that one could protect against the deadly smallpox infection by inoculating the patient with cowpox, an agent that causes a benign infection in humans. A second approach is based on killing the pathogen by mild heat or chemical treatments that do not destroy its characteristic structure. Alternatively, the parts of the pathogen that the immune system learns to recognize can be synthesized or mimicked by the newer techniques of molecular biology and immunology, without the risks involved in introducing a complete pathogen. Finally, it is sometimes possible to produce highly mutant strains of pathogens which cannot cause disease but have essentially the same antigenic composition as the virulent forms. Such strains are used in "live" virus vaccines, like the Sabin polio vaccine, and have the advantage that immunity to the targeted pathogen gets regularly boosted by the periodic growth of the resident vaccine population.

What are the prospects for an AIDS vaccine? It is now well established that the body does mount an immune response upon infection by HIV. Killer T cells that will attack HIV-infected cells as well as antibodies against a number of virus components can be demonstrated in the bloodstream of infected persons. Clearly, in the normal course of events this response is inadequate or is directed against inappropriate determinants, because in a large fraction of cases, infected individuals suffer progressively diminished immune capacity. These observations, which are well documented, have led some researchers to question whether vaccination will ever be effective against HIV. They suggest that this is, after all, a virus that has evolved precisely to be "immune" to the immune system.

Those who see possibilities in the vaccination approach point out that so far HIV has had the luxury of confronting an immune system that had not been primed to lay aside stocks of HIV-specific B and T cells. Vaccination prior to infection could, they suggest, tip the balance in favor of resistance. In support of their view they point to a curious observation that has been made in AIDS patients. HIV-1 is the most rapidly varying animal virus known, and there is often variation from virus isolate to virus isolate. Researchers have examined virus isolated from individuals who have had a large number of potentially infectious contacts—as many as one thousand homosexual encounters over a five-year period. The striking finding was that virus isolated from such individuals showed that in each case the individuals had been infected by only one strain. Even though they were undoubtedly exposed to a variety of strains, late arrivals were unable to gain a foothold in a person who was already infected.

In the hope that vaccination before or even in the early stages after infection may be protective against progress to AIDS, there is a high level of activity in academic, governmental, and industrial laboratories to develop vaccines of one sort or another. There are immunologists who feel that an appropriately killed virus will make the best vaccine. Those critical of the killed virus approach caution that one would be reluctant to inject healthy uninfected individuals with a virus such as HIV, which is characterized by a long latency. How long can we be sure a "dead" virus will remain dead? they ask. To avoid the perils and expense of using whole virus as a vaccinating agent, some groups have turned to genetic engineering techniques to produce parts of the virus that may be able to raise immunity. Another tack being taken is the genetic modification of other viruses such as vaccinia, the harmless agent now used to vaccinate against smallpox, so that these will express components of HIV.

Whatever the routes taken, they all lead to testing in a suitable experimental animal model, a necessary way station along the road to the development of any vaccine. This is necessary to evaluate the safety of a potential vaccine and to gain some knowledge of its most efficacious use. Unfortunately, HIV will not infect the usual battery of species—mice, rats, and guinea pigs—used for medical research. This virus grows only in humans and chimpanzees. Aside from being expensive and difficult to rear, chimpanzees are an endangered species and there are just not enough of them around to support an aggressive program of vaccine testing. Consequently, a great deal of effort is being invested in the search for a suitable alternative, for, whatever clever and ingenious approaches to vaccination are worked out, their development will be seriously bottlenecked until the quest for a practical animal model turns up something suitable.

Thinking About Anti-HIV Drugs

Every now and then there is an opportunity to see Edward G. Robinson on late-night TV in an old black-and-white movie playing Paul Ehrlich, a turn-of-the-century figure who was one of the pioneering giants of immunology and pharmacology. Robinson's Ehrlich is an intense and dedicated researcher who is obsessed with finding a drug that will cure syphilis, in some ways the AIDS of another era. He describes the object of his quest as a "magic bullet," a drug that will be exquisitely selective in its action, killing the deadly bacteria that cause syphilis but leaving the patient's system untouched. Neat trick. This is the holy grail of all drug development programs. The ideal drug is one that conforms perfectly to the principle of selective toxicity, which means that the drug exerts a lethal effect on the pathogen without any ill effects for the host. This obviously desirable goal is seldom achieved in real life. Often there is a similarity between essential metabolic activities that must be conducted by the host and the processes targeted in the pathogen.

Consider the chemotherapy of cancer. Cancer cells are rogue cells that divide without limit, body cells that have become pathological. Anti-tumor drugs are designed to halt cancer's progress by stopping cell division. Since the indispensable multiplication of normal cells uses the same metabolic pathways as does the division of tumor cells, the unavoidable cost of chemotherapy is some damage to normal tissues. A drug directed at a particular pathogen may also have unforeseen and unwanted side effects on host systems, effects that are totally unrelated to the targeted process. Pentamidine is an effective agent for the treatment of *Pneumocystis carinii* pneumonia, but its use can cause a life-threatening rapid fall in blood pressure as well as a fall in blood sugar levels. Furthermore, more often than not, drugs undergo chemical modification as a by-product of normal metabolic processes, and even though the drug itself may have no ill effects, its metabolically altered forms may very well produce unwanted side effects. Penicillin, an almost perfect antibiotic, undergoes modifications that allow it to react with some proteins, producing severe allergies in some people.

For all these reasons, coming up with an effective, safe antiviral drug is a difficult assignment. Viruses, after all, do make a living by substantial use of host cell machinery and host resources. An antiviral "magic bullet" must be aimed with an accuracy that would be daunting even to William Tell. It is not surprising that the hundreds of known antimicrobial drugs in the pharmacologists' larder contrast sharply with the mere half dozen or so antiviral drugs in clinical use.

An antiviral drug might affect the course of a viral infection at any one of the obligatory steps of the virus life cycle. Such a drug might:

- Inactivate the virus before it attaches to a host cell.
- Prevent the virus from attaching to its receptor on the cell or from entering the cell.
- Prevent the viral genetic information from being transferred from the virus to the cell.
- Block the reproduction of the viral genetic information.
- Stop fabrication of virus particles and their exit from infected cells.

Nature has already discovered how to block some of these steps of the virus life cycle. Antibodies specific for the infecting virus will bind to virus particles and mark them for elimination. Some of these antibodies will bind to the specific part of the virus that is designed to attach to receptors on the host cell and thereby block infection. Killer T cells can recognize infected cells and kill them before they have an opportunity to produce virus, thereby thwarting viral replication and assembly. The production of interferon is yet another trick the host defense system has against viruses. When cells are infected by viruses they produce a protein, known as interferon, which acts as an antiviral hormone to inhibit the reproduction of viruses in neighboring cells. Thus even though one cell in a group may die of a viral infection, it manufactures and exports interferon which can protect its neighbors from a similar fate.

What can the pharmaceutical industry provide for the many HIV-infected individuals who will be failed by natural defense mechanisms? Azidodeoxythymidine (AZT) is the first drug to show proven efficacy in the treatment of AIDS. It works by blocking the synthesis of DNA by the AIDS virus. Available by prescription since March 1987, AZT slows virus reproduction and consequently slows its progression through the immune system. Unfortunately, since it interferes with host as well as virus-directed DNA synthesis, AZT is not a therapeutic magic bullet. It can depress the synthesis of red and white blood cells by the bone marrow, and its use must be discontinued in those patients for whom the degree of inhibition becomes life-threatening. In spite of its side effects and even though it does not cure AIDS, it brings the infection under control for a period of time and thereby extends life and improves its quality. As might be expected, the success of AZT has spurred intense research and development to devise other drugs that will inhibit the replication of HIV. The aim is to discover new drugs or to devise combinations of established drugs that either alone or in combination with AZT will produce the same or greater therapeutic effects with less severe side effects. These combinations in turn increase the probability that drugs such as AZT can be used earlier and for longer periods, not only postponing death in those already ill but postponing immune system collapse and progression to full-blown AIDS.

Recognizing that any agent that interferes with DNA synthesis carries the possibility of producing a serious depression in the supply of red and white blood cells, researchers have also paid attention to the development of therapies that will stimulate the body to produce more blood cells. Recent developments in genetic engineering have made it possible to clone the gene for two hormone-like substances that induce the bone marrow to increase its production of blood cells. One of these, GM-CSF, stimulates the development of many types of white blood cells while the other, erythropoietin, dramatically increases the production of red blood cells. There is great hope that therapies employing these natural regulatory substances will make it possible to compensate, at least partially, for the most serious side effects of AZT and its likely successors.

A great deal of thought is also being devoted to how other natural factors such as interferons and interleukins might be used to stimulate or restore immune function that has been compromised by HIV infection. Considerable attention is being given to the question of whether treatment with such immunoregulatory agents will restore sufficient vigor to the immune system to enable it to fight off opportunistic infections. At this writing, the exploration of these possibilities is just beginning, and only time will tell whether these immunoregulatory approaches will be successful. Whatever effective therapies prove successful, it is likely that not one but a combination of therapeutic agents will be required for the effective management of HIV infection and its consequences.

6

A CLINICAL VIEW

OF AIDS

■

THERE IS AN OLD STORY about a group of blind men and an elephant in which each man, because he tactilely explores a different part of the animal, comes away with a different conception of the whole. And so it is with AIDS. The focus on a particular manifestation of AIDS can obscure an appreciation of the fact that this plague is really not a single entity but a state that entertains the possibility of many different diseases. What most of these diseases have in common is that their manifestation in a particular individual requires severe compromise of the immune system. The task is not to describe a single disease "elephant," but to try, with eyes hooded by incomplete or sometimes confusing information, to see a debilitating and life-threatening menagerie of maladies. Clearly, there is not a unitary and common AIDS experience; there is a broad range of AIDS experiences. We should be aware too that the visitation of these experiences is not intrinsically limited to a few currently afflicted groups—homosexual men, certain populations of Africa, and intravenous drug users. Any population whose behavior provides a niche for HIV is a stage on which the different acts of the AIDS tragedy may play.

Who Is at Risk of Experiencing AIDS?

Anyone who suffers infection with HIV is at risk of developing full-blown AIDS. Since the cells that are susceptible to infection lie within the body, any activity—conventional or unconventional, legal or illegal, restorative or destructive, loving or malevolent—that results in the transfer, directly or indirectly, of virus into the bloodstream or inner confines of the body can cause infection. For reasons that will become apparent, the following groups are particularly at risk for HIV infection: homosexual and bisexual males, intravenous drug users, heterosexual partners (male and female) of HIV-infected persons, recipients of blood transfusions, hemophiliacs, and babies gestated in HIV-infected mothers. The risk of each of these groups arises from its exposure to one of the three most important modes of transmission of this virus from one person to another: sexual intercourse; the deliberate or unintended transfer of blood or blood products from an infected to a non-infected person; and maternal infection of offspring during gestation and birth.

Virus particles can be detected in many of the tissues and secretions of those who are infected, but the vast majority of HIV infections can be traced to heterosexual or homosexual intercourse, certainly the most widespread form of intimate human contact. The spread of the virus through communities in several areas of Africa and the documented cases of male-to-female and female-to-male transmission in Europe and the United States establish heterosexual intercourse as a proven vehicle for HIV transmission. The fact that thus far the majority of cases of AIDS in the United States and Europe have been diagnosed in homosexual or bisexual men shows that the deposition of semen during anal intercourse is also an effective means of spreading the virus. The receipt of a transfusion of blood or plasma from an infected person or the sharing of a needle or syringe that has been contaminated by infected blood is an even more effective means of contracting the virus. Before the technology necessary to test blood for HIV contamination was put in place in 1985, receiving a transfusion was a high-risk activity, just as the communal use of injection paraphernalia in a heroin shooting gallery continues to be. Similarly, hemophiliacs who require Factor VIII, a substance isolated from blood plasma that promotes blood clotting, were at great risk of infection until the development in 1984 of a production technology that eliminates HIV from clotting factor preparations. Iatrogenic AIDS, contracted as the unforeseen by-product of restorative therapy, has killed just as effectively as AIDS acquired by venereal or illegal acts.

A quantitative look at who has had AIDS shows that the distribution is far from uniform no matter how the populations examined are indexed. As of December 1988, 132,976 full-blown cases worldwide had been reported to the World Health Organization (WHO). However, due to underreporting, which is in some cases inadvertent and sometimes deliberate, WHO has concluded that this figure is far too low and estimates that the actual number of cases is around 350,000. Of the officially reported cases, most were in the United States (80,538), sub-Saharan Africa (20,905), and Europe (16,883). Elsewhere in the Americas there have been significant concentrations in Brazil and in some parts of the Caribbean. By contrast, Asia and the Pacific Basin report only 1,465 cases, a significant fraction of which have been in Australia.

The distribution of AIDS by behavioral group is quite different in Africa, where the disease primarily affects heterosexuals and cases are equally distributed between men and women, and in the industrialized countries, where homosexual men and I-V drug users are the largest patient groups.

At the beginning of 1989, the breakdown of AIDS cases in the United States by transmission categories was as follows: 60.8 percent homosexual or bisexual male; 19.5 percent I-V drug users; 7.1 percent homosexual male I-V drug users; 4.3 percent heterosexual; 3.4 percent transfusion recipient or hemophiliac; 1.6 percent pediatric; and 3.3 percent undetermined. With respect to racial or ethnic distribution, it is a disease found primarily in whites (58 percent of all cases), blacks (26 percent of all cases), and Hispanic populations (15 percent of all cases). But the distributions in these populations is far from uniform, for the majority of AIDS in whites is found in homosexual males and the larger fraction of black and Hispanic cases can be traced to I-V drug use. Furthermore, even within these groups, the distribution is uneven. Every survey of sexual behavior would lead one to believe that white homosexual males are widely distributed in the United States, but the overwhelming majority of the AIDS in this behavioral category can be traced to just a few major metropolitan areas, with the list headed by New York, San Francisco, and Los Angeles. Again, although the majority of the black population does not live in the New York–northern New Jersey corridor, more than half of the black AIDS patients are found there. Similar considerations hold for the various Hispanic groups. Parts of Florida, the New York area, and Puerto Rico account for most of the caseload, but many of the Hispanic populations of the United States are centered outside these areas.

What these focal numbers tell us is that AIDS incidence is highly dependent on behavior within interacting groups. It does not preferentially infect homosexuals, but it is likely to spread in homosexual communities that have a lifestyle of frequent sex with many different partners, such as the gay New York and San Francisco of the 1970s and early 1980s. AIDS is not a disease with a proclivity for black or Hispanic T cells, but it is likely to spread rapidly in situations where people transfer blood from one to the other such as in the I-V drug-using subcultures of the New York area. Both the individuals and the behaviors have to be transferred to invade another area.

And what figures will the future bring? The year 1991

is common in writings on AIDS because a series of five-year projections were made in 1986. These estimates suggest that by 1991 there may be as many as three million AIDS cases worldwide, but this figure will only be a moment in a continuing tide. Focusing on the problem in a single country, the Centers for Disease Control estimates that the cumulative number of afflicted persons in the United States will rise from nearly 65,000 at mid-1988 to 285,000 in 1991. While the 1980s were a time of AIDS discovery and naïveté, the world of the 1990s will be a widely, deeply, and wearily sophisticated one.

Infection

The experience of AIDS begins like a simple virus infection, with the immune system mobilizing to control it. Then the virus enters a period of latency frequently lasting seven to ten years, safely established in the cells of the immune system. Through time, however, as its presence increases in the body, the same kinds of symptoms may recur in more severe forms over a longer period, the side effects of the body's effort to restore health. For most people a new round of symptoms begins when the immune system has been compromised and the experience of AIDS becomes the experience of the side effects of HIV infection—a host of opportunistic infections, most of which, in the absence of the vulnerability created by HIV, are benign and responsive to therapy.

The specific experiences that follow immediately after infection do not produce a uniform clinical picture. Some patients report no initial symptoms while others experience a period of minor illness marked by fever, a feeling of fatigue and listlessness, loss of appetite, headache and nausea, not unlike the onset of a minor flu. This illness may last from a few days to two weeks or so, and then the person feels better and remains free of symptoms for weeks, months, or even years. Others may experience early episodes of neurologic illness marked by such symptoms as mental deficit, weakness, and sensory loss. In many cases these initial neurological symptoms spontaneously disappear. The time of onset of these symptoms also varies. Some clinicians report a period of three to six weeks between the presumed infecting exposure and the appearance of symptoms, but in one widely cited case, illness developed within six days of a single act of receptive anal intercourse which took place after a long period of abstinence.

In most cases, the clinician finds it difficult to get an accurate fix on the precise date of infection and the first appearance of symptoms. The infecting episode or episodes usually must be determined retrospectively; people rarely have accurate memories of all dates and circumstances of possible exposure, including every sexual or drug connection, and even if they did, they might not report them truthfully. There is also the strong likelihood that many will ignore the first symptoms or mistake them for something else. The picture becomes even more of a montage when one considers that many clinicians believe that a significant fraction of infected individuals in fact show no initial symptoms. Obviously, in the face of such a great degree of variability, one cannot rely solely on the presence or absence of a particular set of symptoms to decide whether infection has taken place. Laboratory confirmation is essential.

The Road to AIDS

The progress from initial infection to severe illness is sometimes very rapid, especially in transfusion cases, but the common occurrence of a gap between the symptoms that follow infection and a slowly rising new tide of problems makes it possible to separate them conceptually. Many of those who travel the road to AIDS encounter the same landmarks along the way, but at first these are simply the familiar signs of the immune system's effort to restore normalcy, appearing in persistent and exaggerated forms. They include fever, fatigue, copious night sweats, and swollen lymph nodes. Actually, any of these symptoms can occur as a consequence of viral or bacterial infection or may accompany certain types of cancer, but when they are chronic and generalized they can be seen as harbingers of AIDS.

Thus, the appearance and persistence for weeks of swollen lymph nodes in two or more areas of the body (excluding the groin) is formally labeled *lymphadenopathy* and is regarded as a probable precursor of AIDS. Rapid weight loss—ten pounds or more over the course of a few weeks that cannot be attributed to exercise or deliberate dieting—is similarly a cause for concern, for although it may signal any one of a broad range of problems such as hormonal imbalance, emotional disturbance, or malignancy, it is often associated with other symptoms in this list during the early stages of AIDS. In Africa, weight loss is so conspicuous that AIDS is called "slim disease." Profound and persistent tiredness not readily attributable to identifiable physical or emotional stress is another symptom frequently reported.

These symptoms are grouped as ARC—AIDS Related Complex—and suggest a losing struggle to maintain homeostasis. Other early symptoms that appear as the immune system is progressively disabled can be recognized as the vanguard of opportunistic infections, illnesses caused by microbes commonly found in the body or the environment that rarely cause disease in people with healthy immune systems. The progressive failure of the immune system opens the way for a variety of lurking pathogens to flourish and manifest themselves as disease. Thrush, a creamy white coating that covers all or part of the tongue, traceable to the yeast *Candida*, is one of the relatively manageable illnesses seen early and often in AIDS patients. A different yeast, *Cryptococcus*, normally harbored by pigeons, causes a much more widely disseminated and life-threatening infection in immunodeficient persons. A persistent cough and progressive shortness of breath that is not associated with vigorous physical activity often signal infection by *Pneu-*

mocystis carinii, a little protozoan that is responsible for the AIDS-related pneumonia, which in a number of cases first prompts the HIV-infected person to seek medical attention.

Full-Blown AIDS

While the term *AIDS* is used popularly to refer to all stages of HIV infection, it technically applies only to the condition following the disabling of the immune system and characterized by opportunistic infections. AIDS confronts the medical arts with an extremely broad and dynamic range of maladies. The physician's response to the challenge is impressive but, with the tools currently available, a losing battle. Just as Hercules found that the Hydra could not be defeated by cutting off one or two of its many heads, treating one of the several manifestations of AIDS does not restore health because a defective immune system, the fundamental lesion of this syndrome, goes unrepaired. The door is thus left open to an endless parade of debilitating and life-threatening infections.

Viruses are well represented in this parade. Taken together, Hepatitis B virus and the Herpes family of viruses are responsible for many of the most severe viral complications of AIDS. Hepatitis B attacks the liver, a key organ often referred to as the body's biochemist because it conducts a wide and critical range of essential activities, including the manufacture of blood-clotting factors, the detoxification of drugs and alcohol, and nutrient processing. Consequently, severe Hepatitis B infection, which greatly diminishes liver function, will have grave consequences for the patient. This liver-destroying virus is found in blood, semen, and saliva and is spread by blood transfusion, sharing of needles, and intimate sexual contact. Since the same behaviors that are responsible for the transmission of HIV also disseminate Hepatitis B, it is not surprising that AIDS patients are often infected with this virus.

The Herpes group encompasses a large number of different viruses, four of which are of particular importance in the pathogenesis of many AIDS cases: Herpes simplex I and II, Epstein-Barr virus (EBV), and Cytomegalovirus (CMV). An important aspect of the biology of all of these viruses is illustrated by the answer to the locker room question, "What's the difference between love and herpes?" to which sophisticates reply, "Herpes is forever." Like HIV, each has the insidious capacity to integrate its genetic material into the genetic machinery of the cells it infects. In this way it can maintain a lifetime residency in the host, producing intermittent periods of disease separated by long periods of latency.

The specific disease effects produced by various Herpesviruses are as diverse as the viruses themselves. A much-discussed member of this family, HSV II, is the causative agent of the sexually transmitted disease "herpes," referred to above, which is characterized by the production of lesions on the genitals. It is a common infection of AIDS patients, and often also presents as painful lesions around the nose, mouth, or anus. In AIDS patients it is progressive and can be very severe if it fails to respond to treatment. Epstein-Barr virus, the agent responsible for mononucleosis, the familiar "kissing disease" that frequents college campuses, is extremely widespread, and a large fraction of the world's population has been exposed to it—perhaps as many as 80 percent of us have antibodies to EBV, including almost all homosexual AIDS patients. Some clinicians have suggested that there may be a causal relationship between the relatively high incidence of B-cell cancer (*B lymphoma*) and the reactivation of latent EBV in these immunocompromised patients. The last Herpesvirus mentioned, CMV, in addition to invading a number of internal organs including the adrenal glands, liver, and colon, can also infect the eyes and result in partial or even complete blindness.

It is not surprising that bacterial infections are often a significant part of the AIDS clinical experience. The same bacterial pneumonias traceable to *Streptococcus pneumoniae*, and *Hemophilus influenzae* that affect the general population occur with greater frequency in AIDS patients. Tired and nearly defeated old warhorses like tuberculosis are again off and running, particularly among patients whose AIDS is traceable to I-V drug use or patients born in areas where TB is endemic, such as Haiti or other areas of the Caribbean. The *Salmonella* bacteria that are frequent contaminants of poultry and cause more than a million cases of stomach disorders a year in the population of the United States, can produce severe diarrhea whose effects are exacerbated in immunodeficient persons. In addition to the familiar panoply of bacterial infections, some very unfamiliar bacterial infections are appearing in AIDS patients, one of which is traceable to a widely distributed bacterial complex, *Mycobacterium avium-intracellulare*. This complex causes a tuberculosis-like illness which may appear in the lungs but is not limited to that organ and tends to spread to other sites in the body such as the liver, bone marrow, and gastrointestinal tract. It is a devastating infection and cause for the gravest concern in the immuno-compromised.

Microbes of one sort or another are not the only problems encountered by AIDS patients. In ways that are not completely understood, the immune system provides the body's major defense against the growth of tumors. It has long been known that individuals such as transplant patients, whose immune systems are deliberately suppressed to prevent organ rejection, are at greater risk for cancer than people with fully functional immunity. Therefore, it is not surprising that cancer is all too frequently diagnosed in persons with AIDS. Although many AIDS patients die from the unchecked onslaught of wave after wave of microbial infections, others fall victim to the growth of tumors or a combination of the effects of both.

A number of tumors seen in AIDS patients have their origin in the lymphoid system, including the B-cell lymphomas. Another type of cancer, Kaposi sarcoma, which is otherwise quite rare, is seen in a large number of AIDS cases, but its distribution among different groups of patients is noteworthy. In the United States this cancer, which is characterized by dark brown or purplish nodules and patches on the skin but also attacks and destroys organs internally, is found in almost a third of the gay men who develop AIDS. In Africa, it is seen in heterosexual men as well as in women and children. On the other hand, fewer than 1 in 20 intravenous drug users with AIDS develops Kaposi sarcoma. An understanding of the mechanisms responsible for the puzzling differences in the incidence of this type of tumor in different groups might provide important clues to its genesis.

But the band does indeed play on, and yet another dimension of risk is opened when the central nervous system plays host to HIV. Viral damage erodes the system's capacity to exercise the precise coordination and control that is indispensable for such ordinary miracles as walking. There is also memory loss and, not uncommonly, a syndrome of mental confusion and derangement. In fact, this progressive AIDS dementia is ultimately suffered by as many as a third of all AIDS patients and can be traced to the direct and indirect effects of HIV infection on brain tissue. AIDS-associated damage to the spinal cord is responsible for a variety of neuromuscular malfunctions, including varying degrees of weakening or paralysis in the lower extremities and loss or impairment of muscle coordination.

Unsettling as this synopsis of the consequences of HIV infection may be, it fails to express the way in which this long list of afflictions can converge on the individual patient. One way to get a sense of that multiple convergence is to look at a formal case history in which the physician summarizes in terse and technical language months of suffering and fear experienced by the unnamed patient and months of effort to understand and respond. The following case study has been adapted from the pages of a leading medical journal. A stark way of presenting the experience of an individual, this account is as unsatisfying in its own way as the list of opportunistic infections or the statistics of AIDS in different regions, but it reveals an essential dimension of the story, abstracting the medical detail from the personal tragedy. It was not possible to have a true sense of the enormity of the Holocaust without a confrontation with images of bodies stacked like cordwood, and somehow we must combine an awareness of AIDS in terms of thousands of faceless victims with the sense of medical detail as well as individual stories. Gradually more and more Americans will supplement the eloquent personal stories they have read with the face of a member of their family or of someone from their high school class or their office or neighborhood.

A Case Study of AIDS Dementia

A twenty-eight-year-old homosexual man contracted *Pneumocystis carinii* pneumonia in 1982. Subsequently, his clinical course was complicated by recurrent perianal [around the anus] Herpes simplex infection, central nervous system toxoplasmosis [infection with the parasitic protozoan *Toxoplasma gondii*], and disseminated *Mycobacterium avium-intracellulare* and Cytomegalovirus infections. He also had intestinal cryptosporidiosis [infection with the diarrhea-causing protozoan *Cryptosporidium*] which resulted in Vitamin B_{12} deficiency. Gradual onset of gait disturbance occurred in October 1984. This progressed to paraplegia [paralysis of the lower limbs], with urinary and fecal incontinence over the next three months. In January 1985, the patient was hospitalized for these problems. Physical examination was notable for severe lower extremity weakness, abnormal sense of position in the toes, and dementia. A CAT scan demonstrated marked cerebral atrophy and hydrocephalus [accumulation of fluid on the brain]. A spinal tap was performed and examination of the cerebrospinal fluid obtained was unremarkable and cultures were negative for bacteria and fungi. However, a culture of cerebrospinal fluid was positive for HIV. The patient's course deteriorated and he died in March 1985. Postmortem examination of the nervous system showed microglia [a type of cell found in the nervous system] nodule formation, and demyelination [loss of the nerve's insulating sheath] in the cerebrum. In addition, a lymphoma [a cancer of the lymphatic system] was found in the left occipital [back of the skull] region. Specimens obtained from the frontal lobe of the brain and spinal cord twenty-four hours after death also yielded HIV when cultured.

[Adapted from David Ho et al., *New England Journal of Medicine* 313 (1985): 1493–97.]

■

The brief sentences of the medical case report omit much of the story of this one man's experience, but even without a face or a name it is possible to sense some of the texture of a life and its unraveling. We hear nothing here of early symptoms, but we can infer from the variety of sexually transmitted diseases that this man was a participant in an urban gay community, perhaps an experience of emancipation, perhaps also of fulfilling love. By 1982, when he was diagnosed, he would have begun to see friends dying and to feel mounting anxiety at the mysterious illness around him, and perhaps to connect it with fatigue or sleepless nights of his own. He was diagnosed and hospitalized with *Pneumocystis*, experiencing progressive and increasing difficulty in breathing. We can guess that after the *Pneumocystis* was diagnosed and treated, he was able to go home and probably able to return to work for a period of time, with diverse and steadily increasing medical problems, episodes of hope and improvement and episodes of despair. We are not told the other circumstances of his life, whether he had adequate financial resources or became rapidly destitute when he was unable to work, whether his family supported him or, like many families of AIDS patients, refused to see him. In any case, his condition continued to deteriorate. By 1984, he was unable to control his lower body and to function on his own, suffering a complication of AIDS that was just beginning to be recognized, neurological deterioration, a mystery within a mystery which test after test failed to explain. Part of the agony of AIDS is that even when you have been diagnosed with the syndrome, the day-to-day experience is opaque. When he was hospitalized an array of tests, including such painful measures as a spinal tap, failed at first to identify the cause of his neurological symptoms. Throughout the course of his illness we can imagine a gathering darkness, a fluctuation between fear and transient hope, between rage and depression. Many patients with AIDS dementias experience periods of confusion and agitation, gradually becoming mute and ceasing to respond.

"When I lie down," said Job, "I say, When shall I arise, and the night be gone? and I am full of tossings to and fro unto the dawning of the day. My flesh is clothed with worms and clods of dust; my skin is broken, and become loathsome. My days are swifter than a weaver's shuttle, and are spent without hope" (Job 7:4–6). Behind every AIDS statistic there are thousands of such case reports and records. Behind every such record there are hundreds of hours of unrecorded pain.

Therapy

At present, there is no cure for the immunodeficiency that is responsible for AIDS and no way of arresting the attack of the AIDS virus on the nervous system. Full-blown AIDS is still uniformly fatal. Because AIDS opens the door for a diverse and dynamic spectrum of diseases, there is also no single "off-the-rack" therapy for its clinical management. Each patient requires a tailor-made therapeutic approach that will need frequent and sometimes radical alteration. If the patient's disease spectrum includes cancer, then the usual tools of the oncologist— radiation, chemotherapy, and surgery—will be brought to bear. Most cases will require that a great deal of attention be given to the management of one or sometimes two or more infectious diseases occurring and recurring in different rhythms. The usually complex juggle of therapies is sometimes further complicated by the conflicting nature of the mix.

Anti-tumor chemotherapy is inherently immunosuppressive because it tends to inhibit the cell division necessary for whatever cells of the patient's immune system remain to mount defensive responses. AIDS patients are weakened patients who in many cases have to withstand the side effects of some of the most debilitating drugs available to medical science. In most AIDS cases, rest and restorative therapy rather than the assault of an ensemble of powerful drugs would be called for were it not for the clear and inescapably grave consequences of allowing a fulminating infection or a spreading tumor to go unchecked. The irony of treating AIDS patients is that powerful and effective curative therapies are no more than symptomatic treatments for them, temporary palliatives, for this is a disease whose symptoms are themselves diseases.

The list of drugs prescribed for AIDS patients is even more dauntingly polysyllabic than the list of pathogens that afflict them, and the examples presented here represent no more than a sampling of current therapy which is constantly undergoing revision. A variety of powerful antibiotics are available for the treatment of bacterial infections. Members of the penicillin family, such as ampicillin, are often quite effective against *Salmonella* and many strains of *Streptococcus* and *Staphylococcus*, and they are relatively free of serious side effects in those not allergic to them, but there are many bacterial infections that are commoner in AIDS patients against which the penicillins are not effective. Infections with the *Mycobacterium avium-intracellulare* complex have been very difficult to control with antibiotic therapy, and there is an active search for a drug or combination of drugs that will bring this opportunistic infection under control. In treating some bacterial infections that are not sensitive to penicillin, other powerful but potentially damaging antibiotics are often employed, such as chloramphenicol, which suppresses the production of both red and white blood cells, or gentamicin, which is damaging to the kidneys and can cause deafness.

There are several drugs (pentamidine or the combination TMP and SMZ) that can be used in the treatment of *Pneumocystis carinii*, the most common opportunistic agent in AIDS patients in the United States, and in preventing recurrences. Fungal infections, such as those of the yeast *Candida*, are difficult to cure completely and tend to recur. With luck, some cases can be brought under initial control with such orally administered antifungal drugs as Nystatin or clotrimazole, which are free of serious side effects, but more stubborn initial episodes or relapsing cases may require the use of ketoconazole, a drug that may damage the liver, or amphotericin B, which is toxic to the kidneys and may produce other side effects as well. Central nervous system infection with *Cryptococcus*, another yeast mentioned earlier, is life-threatening and must be addressed with drugs such as amphotericin B.

Viruses present a particular problem to the management of infection by drug therapy because the number of effective antiviral agents is quite small compared to the great variety of viral agents known to cause disease. Nevertheless there are drugs, such as Acyclovir, that in some cases have been useful in treating Herpes simplex and Herpes zoster. Another drug, DHPG, has shown promise for the treatment of Cytomegalovirus.

The therapy of AIDS is very much like that of tuberculosis before the advent of curative antibiotic therapies. Until the 1950s, doctors were limited to treating the superficial manifestations of severe infection with *Mycobacterium tuberculosis*, the agent responsible for TB. The introduction of the drug Isoniazid, and soon after of other effective antibiotics such as rifampin, made it possible to eliminate the pathogen and thus actually cure the disease. There are clear parallels in this experience for AIDS. Until it is possible to eliminate or control HIV and to restore immunocompetence to AIDS patients, there will be no cure for AIDS, only palliative treatment of the consequences of the fundamental lesion in the body's capacity to protect itself.

Until such a therapeutic restoration can be effected, the role of clinicians should be to use available tools to make the lot of the patient as comfortable as possible. This is not always done. Aside from the considered application of appropriate medical technology, therapy should recognize the importance of emotional support and the maintenance of patient dignity. Both these ends are likely to be well served by sparing the patient the trauma of painful and exhausting diagnostic procedures or heroic and debilitating therapies that hold little hope for meaningful improvements in well-being.

7

TO KNOW

OR NOT TO KNOW

■

ONE OF THE FIRST significant developments that followed the discovery of HIV was the development of a blood test for HIV-1, the most common member of the HIV family. Undergoing such a test is an AIDS experience that will certainly be shared by millions, and there are already a variety of testing programs in place. The test for the AIDS virus, like the virus itself, is becoming a fact of life, one that is potentially pathological unless we find appropriate ways to manage it, and one that can be expected to cause recurrent debates between those who advocate coercive testing, testing "hawks," and testing "doves," who believe all diagnostic testing should be elective. It is almost as important to understand the limitations and social implications of testing as it is to understand the virus itself and its clinical manifestations.

The blood testing procedures currently in use for HIV are based on the fact that infection with a virus does not go unnoticed by the immune system, which manufactures antibodies able to bind to a number of the virus's protein components. These telltale antibodies eventually appear in the blood serum of most infected persons, and it is the presence of antibodies—not virus—that is usually tested. The antibodies are highly specific and so, as a result, are the tests. Tests for HIV-1 do not sensitively determine the presence or absence of infection with HIV-2, although HIV-2, like other perturbations in the immune system, may sometimes affect test results. This means that new tests will have to be developed as new types of HIV emerge and begin to spread. That they will do so seems probable, for the HIV family of viruses appears to be capable of rapid genetic variation.

There are two common approaches to testing, each of which relies on confronting a small blood sample with a trace of virus and looking for recognition: ELISA (an acronym for enzyme-linked immunoassay), the simpler and cheaper of the two, and the Western blot. No one who has ever stood in a reception line will be surprised that recognition is not an infallible process. A negative ELISA indicates that antibodies capable of responding to HIV have not been detected in the patient's blood sample, and the patient is said to be *seronegative*. On the other hand, a positive ELISA asserts that the patient does have HIV-reactive antibodies and contingent on confirmation by further testing, the person may be judged *seropositive* and is said to have *seroconverted*.

This is one case where a technical term, such as seroconversion, is useful as a reminder of the need for further interpretation. Seroconversion takes time. With HIV, the process typically takes about six weeks after the virus enters the body, and may take as long as six months or more. Occasionally it never occurs at all, even when the individual has developed full-blown AIDS. The term *infection*, by contrast, refers to an event that presumably occurred on a specific date.

Several years ago there was an epidemic of "answer jokes." (Jokes, passed from person to person, move through society very much like epidemics, dying out as we gradually build up resistance to particular forms of humor.) Answer jokes posed riddles such as, "What is

the question to which the answer is Chicken Sukiyaki?"*
The AIDS test is like such riddles. It supplies answers—
but it is not always clear to what question.

How then does a man or woman interpret a negative
ELISA? In the majority of cases a negative test means
that infection has not taken place, but there are really
three possibilities: (1) there is no HIV antibody in the
blood, because HIV has never entered the body; (2) there
is no HIV antibody in the blood—yet—but the virus
has entered the body; or (3) there is HIV antibody in
the blood but the test failed to detect it. No test is
foolproof.

Thus people who have, on a single occasion, tested
negative for HIV-reactive antibodies should not be convinced of their freedom from infection. Even more important, they should not be convinced of their luck or
the safety of their lifestyle. Two or three negative tests,
spaced out over nine months or a year without new or
continuing risky activities, do provide considerable con-
fidence (although not certainty) that infection has not
taken place.

An initially positive ELISA, because of the gravity of
the result, is subject to reexamination. A number of
conditions, including pregnancy and other perturbations
of the immune system (infections, cancers, and so on),
increase the risk of false positives, but the major problem
is simply human error. Additional confirmatory tests are
needed.

A properly performed and confirmed positive test
means that an individual is significantly at risk of eventually developing full-blown AIDS. It does not answer
the question of whether the person will in fact develop
AIDS, although clinical experience has shown that with
each passing year after infection, a further fraction of the
individuals who are seropositive will progress to AIDS.

*The question: "What was the nickname of the only Japanese
kamikaze pilot to survive World War II?"

Thus, a confirmed positive test for HIV is a matter of grave concern and provokes great anxiety. It does not say when or how the person will die. It does not say whether the person is good or bad, innocent or guilty. It probably does answer the question of whether this individual can, under rather narrowly defined circumstances, infect someone else with the virus, but it does not say whether he or she will deal with that possibility responsibly, nor that someone who is uninfected today will be uninfected tomorrow. It does not answer the question of how society should use that information, or who should have access to it. In fact, the implications of the test result are so ambiguous that they should always be accompanied by skilled and knowledgeable counseling. For this reason the home testing kits that will surely become available may do more harm than good. Even when the result is negative, counseling offers an opportunity to discuss risks. When it is determined that an individual carries the AIDS virus, this is the time to teach him or her how to live with it responsibly, perhaps for many years.

Although test results carry a risk of misinformation or psychological damage, there is little reason to question the advisability of testing when an individual or a physician operating within the constraints of the patient-doctor relationship requests the procedure. An individual may feel a psychological need to know, particularly if there are indicators of possible HIV infection, and increasing numbers are haunted by fear of infection even when their lifestyles are relatively risk-free. A physician may find the results of such a test useful in confirming a diagnosis, particularly of an AIDS-related condition. But there are some caveats even here. AIDS testing can be addictive if done repeatedly in a search for security, which the test cannot provide. Individuals who wish to be tested will want to consider alternative testing sites unless they are certain that a clinic or personal physician they may have relied on for a long time is a trustworthy source of well-informed counseling, genuine confidentiality, and sustained commitment to the care of sero-positive patients.

Another function of elective testing may be its use to mark moments of decision. Significant shifts in lifestyle, particularly when they affect relationships or activities supported by well-established habits, are easier to make with some kind of ritual marker. Some people use such rituals as confession and absolution as ways of making a fresh start; others make a ceremony of announcing their resolutions to their friends. A test can also be used as such a marker of resolutions to follow safer sex guidelines.

Still, although there are many reasons for wanting test results, and reassurance is an understandable desire, individuals should be warned not to use negative results as a basis for unsafe behavior. It is not necessary to have reliable, up-to-date knowledge of antibody status in order to enjoy sex safely, but when a man wishes to offer a kidney transplant to his brother, it is important to know whether he has AIDS. When a couple is deciding to have a child, they might wish to do so only if free of infection. But anyone considering an AIDS test should consider in advance what the implications of the result will be. Perhaps it will suggest a behavior change that should be taken in any case, and the test is unnecessary. In general, it is the greater wisdom always to behave as if infection is possible, and to make the taking of precautions a part of normal behavior. The fantasy of using test results to establish risk-free zones of seronegative promiscuity is a dangerous and irrational effort to deny the fact that AIDS has become a part of the world we live in. Still, elective testing, confidentially conducted and accompanied by counseling, though more expensive and invasive, should be as freely available as a blood pressure test.

These are the factors involved in individual decisions on testing, but there are two other testing approaches that need to be understood—testing for epidemiological purposes and compulsory screening.

The development of a version of the ELISA test specific for HIV antibodies was a very important step toward understanding the course of disease in individuals and the pattern of the epidemic. It was the test that made it possible to prove that AIDS was being transmitted through transfusions and blood products, and to force blood banks to change procedures and institute controls, although these are in place only in industrialized countries. It was also the test that made it possible to prove that the dying infants that began to appear in big city hospitals in the early 1980s were suffering from the same disease as adult homosexuals. The tests are not a boon, however, unless we know when to use them and how to use the results, the contexts in which the economic and social costs of testing are likely to be justified by the expected benefits.

There is an interesting parallel between the immune system and society, for clearly the immune system does have the capacity to recognize the virus and to mark cells taken over by the virus—but this capacity does not lead to effective action. The secret of HIV's success once it is disseminated in the body is its inaccessibility; HIV infection is already widely disseminated in the society where coercive testing may tend to increase inaccessibility. This is the phenomenon called "driving the disease underground."

Proposals to legislate mass screening are generally directed at whole categories of persons: marriage-license applicants, prisoners, or residents of particular locations. The arguments are different in different cases, but analysis arrives at a recurrent result: other policies may do more good, do less damage, and cost less. A Harvard University study analyzing the likely consequences of a nationwide program of using the ELISA test to screen marriage-license applicants for HIV antibodies arrived at striking findings. On the basis of the estimated present frequency of HIV infection in the population, these workers could calculate that of the nearly 4 million Americans who marry each year, only a little over 1,300 are actually infected with the AIDS virus. However, since the ELISA test generates some false positives, additional confirmatory testing would have to be done to pick these 1,300 individuals out of the group of around 9,000 initially identified. Furthermore, the costs of such a program would be significant, even for an industrialized nation, while many developing nations have public health budgets that allocate less than the cost of an ELISA test per year to each individual. Each year in the United States over $20 million would have to be paid for the tests alone. The Harvard group estimated that the costs of counseling and administration of such a program would bring the costs up to $100 million annually.

The whole cost is not paid in dollars and cents. The persons falsely identified as positive in the initial ELISA test would pay a high psychological price during the anxious wait for confirmatory results, and some of them might find that they or their intimates remain under a lingering shadow, never fully reassured. Undoubtedly, there would be some canceled weddings and a few suicides. Finally, since there are between one million and two million HIV-infected persons in the United States, this hundred-million-dollar-a-year premarital screening program would detect only around 0.1 percent of the infected total in the population. The benefits are low, the costs are high. Premarital screening is easily proposed because of the historical precedents. It has been a tool in the control of syphilis, but its apparent usefulness has depended on the availability of treatment and on the relatively high proportion of couples that postponed sexual relations until after marriage. The analogy today is false.

Another easy context where there is an historical analogy is the screening of immigrants or visa applicants for such infectious diseases as tuberculosis. It is too late to stop HIV at the border, and it is irresponsible to expel carriers instead of providing education and care, especially to those who may have acquired the infection in this country. Screening visa applicants for HIV would trigger reciprocal controls and discourage trade and tourism, while screening immigrants represents no more than closing the barn door after the horse is stolen. Since the United States has the largest number of reported AIDS cases in the world, it might be more logical, but equally futile, to screen U.S. citizens applying for passports to travel abroad.

In general, the major justification offered for proposals to screen large numbers of people is that the spread of AIDS will be significantly reduced by identifying infected individuals and preventing them from spreading the infection. It would be a mistake to concur on such testing programs without a clear understanding of how the results would be used, of how this prevention would be achieved. Quarantine? Cuba is segregating seropositive individuals in a sanatorium that claims to maintain many of the conditions of normal life. Deportation of noncitizens? This policy is already in place in the Soviet Union. Denial of civil rights? Forced abortion? Or perhaps only education and counseling.

Coercive testing creates the possibility of punishing the victim by stigmatization or even incarceration, rather than giving every member of the society the capacity for self-defense and enlisting the cooperation of the infected group in the effort. The exclusion from the community of those afflicted with a disease is sometimes useful but it carries great risks of injustice. It is not a new idea. In biblical days, there was a great deal of fear associated with skin diseases, leprosy being the central and most terrifying example, and sections of the biblical book of Leviticus read like a diagnostic manual. We are still haunted by echoes of these texts. In them, the early recognition of the value of quarantine is absorbed into a preoccupation with avoiding physical pollution that included menstruating women or women who had recently given birth, and still provides much of the emotional force behind responses to unfamiliar sexual practices and discussions of "bodily fluids." The regulations go on for chapter after chapter. They led to the unnecessary exclusion of many people from full social participation, including people with various transient skin infections. To be classified as a leper was to be "as one dead." Any person seen to have various kinds of rash "is a leprous man, he is unclean: the priest shall pronounce him utterly unclean; his plague is in his head. And the leper in whom the plague is, his clothes shall be rent, and his head bare, and he shall put a covering upon his upper lip, and shall cry, Unclean, unclean. All the days wherein the plague shall be in him he shall be defiled; he is unclean: he shall dwell alone; without the camp shall his habitation be" (Leviticus 13:44–46).

Today we know that leprosy is far less infectious than the ancients believed. The fear of disease is moderated by knowledge and by traditions of compassionate and dedicated care, but in some quarters dedication again seems to be giving way to panic, and AIDS has come to be surrounded with the same aura of fear and horror that once attended leprosy. Under these circumstances, where we are not yet ready to make responsible use of findings, testing can be dangerous rather than beneficial.

Fortunately, given these ambiguities, proposals for mass screening can be rejected on other grounds. Aside from the significant expenditures necessary to find a relatively small fraction of the pool of infected persons, the attempt to identify carriers can produce a false sense of security. It will miss those individuals who are infected but have not yet become seropositive; it will miss those who become infected after they have been tested; it may miss antibodies to new strains of virus; and, because it is not infallible, it will even miss some with AIDS antibodies at the time of testing. Unless coupled with an aggressive (and costly) program of counseling for negative as well as positive testees, people who have tested negative may be tempted to engage in activities that we know will spread the virus. It is one of the paradoxes of this paradoxical plague that testing everyone in Texas or New York and informing them of the results could be a factor in spreading AIDS.

These arguments apply best to mass screening programs, and it is no accident that the Harvard group chose premarital testing as their case study. Programs that concentrate on defined risk groups would of course produce more identifications, but not much new information, since we know already what groups are at risk and the results would still not be accurate person by person. Testing all members of a given risk group is to be preferred only to segregation of all members without testing, an even more drastic form of discrimination.

More seriously, this approach leads to a fixation on risk groups, which is dangerous because the risk groups of today may not be the risk groups of tomorrow, and if all carriers who are risk group members were identified the epidemic would still continue in other groups. We do not need additional screening to know that participants in the urban gay culture of the 1970s are at risk. The danger comes from assuming that only they are at risk.

On the other hand, public health officials do have a critical need to monitor the distribution of the virus in the population. Because of the long latency between infection and the appearance of disease, it is not wise to wait and infer virus distribution by the incidence of full-blown AIDS. By the time disease shows up in a population, the virus may be widespread, and instead of a few infected individuals one is confronted with a latent epidemic. Fortunately, the application of sophisticated sampling and statistical analysis allows an assessment of the frequency of infection in a population category by testing only a few members of that population. Furthermore, since the information is being gathered to find out the status of the epidemic, not whether Mr. Jones or Ms. Day is infected, anonymity is easy to protect. There is no need to identify the samples to be tested by name, only by demographic characteristics that might be useful in planning such as age, sex, occupation, and ethnicity.

Furthermore, the error inherent in the test does not pose the difficulties for population studies that are encountered when one tests individuals diagnostically. Small scientifically selected samples can be used, and the results can simply be corrected for a predictable number of false positives and negatives. Corrected figures can then be compared for different times and settings, and examined to detect changes of only a fraction of a percent in the prevalence of the virus. Public health officials would then know something was afoot and begin to determine the factors responsible for the increase and the appropriate response.

Clearly, survey testing such as that described, where the primary purpose is to establish the distribution of HIV infection and provide an early warning system for the spread of the virus, can be conducted far more cheaply than diagnostic testing. It provides information that can direct educational programs to the appropriate audiences and is an invaluable aid to public health planning and the efficient allocation of public health funds and personnel. Increasingly, surveys of knowledge about AIDS and willingness to take precautions are becoming available. By comparing these to surveys of prevalence, it will be possible to determine when the spread of understanding in a given population begins to outpace the spread of infection.

Some writers have argued that it is unethical to withhold the individual results of such sample testing, but arguably it is unethical to convey them to the individuals without undertaking the expenses of confirmatory laboratory tests and of full counseling and follow-up. The statistical results of screening are genuinely informative and can be used by communities in rational decision making; because the information about individuals is ambiguous, particularly on the basis of single tests, it cannot be used for rational decision making. Information and communication are the keys to controlling the epidemic, but misinformation and miscommunication may do more harm than good.

The process of understanding the meaning of AIDS tests and using them to inform decision making is still in its early stages. Still, we have the test now, and, as with any technological possibility, we must decide what to do with it and what to say to individuals who see in testing a technological "quick fix" and who bring steady pressure for legislation. The hope for a solution through testing is reminiscent of other situations in which it has been tempting to try to resolve problems of social policy with tests or scores whose meanings are not fully understood. The effort to administer schools on the basis of IQ tests, which has the same aura of science and objectivity, is equally ambiguous in the information it provides, and likely to lead to unfairness. Test results are a poor and partial approximation to self-knowledge. The differences in possible outcomes of the testing debate are momentous. At one extreme, there is the possibility of enforced universal testing, used as the criterion for quarantine. At the other extreme, there is the possibility that individual testing can be integrated into a set of policies promoting voluntary responsible behavior.

The situation at the moment is one in which test results can be dangerous—dangerous to the individual because of the discrimination they may trigger, and dangerous to the society because of their ambiguity. Testing may not turn out to be the centerpiece of policy. It may eventually prove easier to persuade most people to practice safe sex and to avoid needle sharing without testing, and this is probably the only way to move in third world countries where testing is clearly a misuse of resources except as a population-monitoring device to advise policy.

Since the tests exist and will be used, the better part of wisdom is to try to arrive at a state where knowledge of the test result is preferable to ignorance even for those who are infected, just as early knowledge of one of the treatable cancers is preferable to ignorance. This means better and cheaper tests, which will surely become available, and a better understanding of their import, which is by no means guaranteed. It is important to think now about how testing programs can be prevented from being destructive. Political climates can change rapidly, and time is already running out for the effort to guarantee confidentiality at the federal level and to protect civil rights. As with the effort to prevent the spread of infection, the effort to prevent injustice is of little use after the fact.

What can be done to make testing programs more beneficial in their effect? At present there are no benefits to the individual from a "positive" test result, except the early replacement of ambiguity by certainty (a preferred state for some people). Early identification, accompanied by counseling and psychological support, must be turned into something desirable. This means controlling negative results such as discrimination, which are currently controlled largely through confidentiality. But confidentiality must be backed up by legal protection and by continuing efforts to convince the public that discrimination is not a measure of reasonable self-defense but an unjustifiable denial of the rights of others, like unjustified discrimination against any group. Because testing provides an opportunity for establishing communication with an individual whose cooperation needs to be enlisted for the safety of others, we would do well to discover or create rewards for voluntary testing. The medical community is beginning to focus on the stage between infection and the onset of severe symptoms—as early as possible—and seeking useful measures to be taken at the onset of swollen glands and night sweats, instead of focusing on the terminal stages. Similarly, a government-supported health and disability insurance scheme could reward early diagnosis with later benefits.

Knowledge always has a cost, is always liable to misuse, always brings a burden of responsibility. The person who knows that he or she is infected with AIDS carries not only the burden of the fear of early death but the burden of protecting others, the knowledge that his or her body can cause death. Testing promises to eliminate ignorant transmission, creating culpability, but it is not clear that those who know they are seropositive will behave more responsibly than those who, uncertain of their antibody status, face a double challenge to protect themselves and to protect others. Country after country and state after state are enacting laws or reinterpreting old laws to make it a criminal act for a person who knowingly carries the AIDS virus to have unprotected sex. Although alcoholism can be regarded as a disease, and drunkenness as a state of diminished responsibility, it is not appropriate to absolve individuals who cause the deaths of others of all responsibility because they are drunk, or to allow the right of privacy to prevent the testing of alcohol levels in the blood.

Above all, we must learn to think of the individuals who live the seropositive life with grace and maturity, learning of their own infection and taking steps not to pass it on with all the realism and self-discipline that this entails, as heroes in this encounter with disease, fighting at the barricades while others move to safety. Many in this group will provide the leadership both in prevention of the epidemic's spread and in care for the afflicted. Learning to value them in their difficult role is part of learning to live with AIDS.

8

PERSONAL

CHOICES

■

IT'S A NEW WORLD, with new risks and new responsibilities. Some of the inventions to be made will be shared by the entire society in the form of new laws and institutions or technological capabilities. Others will be worked out by individuals, piecing together old conventions and new imperatives, trying to hold on to a sense of self and a measure of delight. Scientific progress and political change take time, but it is already time for individuals, sick or well, seropositive or seronegative, to arrive at a personal understanding of the situation and to begin to make the behavioral changes appropriate to living their lives in the new environment. Not everyone has the capacity to make choices, whether because of a lack of knowledge or a lack of resources or a lack of freedom. This book is designed for those who do have that capacity, who will struggle to preserve it by avoiding the servitude of addiction and to increase it by thought and discussion.

The first step is to look around and see who inhabits this new world. Not risk groups and safe groups, for such boundaries are evanescent. Not saints who are uninfected and sinners with AIDS. There are people who know that their behavior puts them at risk and others who know of no present danger. Some are tightly locked into dangerous patterns like intravenous drug use which are almost impossible to escape without help. Others have drifted into habits of casual sex. Some people are already sick, facing a slow and painful death, and yet there are still choices they can make. Others are neighbors or lovers or caretakers of those who are sick. Some people have had the antibody status of their blood tested, with all the uncertainties that implies. Most of those reading this book can make a reasonable estimate of the extent to which they are at risk at this moment, without knowing absolutely whether they are infected. But the logic of the disease and of the uncertainty in which we live is that every individual should act on the possibility that others around them are infected with AIDS—and on the parallel possibility that they themselves carry the virus and have the obligation to protect others. In the context of these two possibilities, the sensible thing is to take realistic precautions, to acquire a high level of behavioral immunity, and to get on with living a rewarding and constructive life. This is a two-sided ethic that depends on both caring for others and caring for oneself. People will often act responsibly for others even when they will not do so for themselves, but at the same time people need to feel good about themselves to care for their own health.

Living with AIDS is a little like applying Kant's categorical imperative—acting as if your behavior were to become a rule for the whole society, affecting you as well as others. It's also somewhat like a version of the Golden Rule worked out to apply to the many situations, like marriage, in which the parties are necessarily different.

In working out how to behave in a world that includes the AIDS virus, driving is a useful analogy. Automobile accidents account for many more deaths in this country every year than AIDS is likely to do unless the epidemic continues unchecked for some time, and yet most people continue to drive. The vast majority of drivers have learned to be concerned for their own safety and for the safety of others as well—in fact, they come to realize that these are inseparable. Most drivers do not follow the rules they have been taught exactly but they do work out their own calibration of risks, going a little over the speed limit sometimes and under it when bad weather increases the danger, putting together a personal style that draws on the example of others and on the public rules and is still an expression of personality. On the road excessive caution can sometimes cause accidents. Increased knowledge, increased control, and uncompromised mental capacity all make driving safer, and most people find positive pleasure in their own competence behind the wheel, for even with the need for careful attention and a life-saving seat belt carefully fastened, driving is an experience of freedom. But to complete the analogy, we have to compare the arrival of the AIDS virus to a change in road conditions sufficient to require a whole new calibration.

The first decision that presents itself to every individual living in this new world is *to behave in such a way as to neither contract nor transmit AIDS*. The behaviors are almost the same, though they can be expressed in elaborate and skillful precautions or by monogamy or total abstinence. The message to individuals must be: "You care about yourself and about other people. You like a good time and you plan ahead to have the good time safely." The difficulty is not so much in defining what is needed as in reshaping one's own behavior patterns. The evidence is in, however, that it can be done. While rates of syphilis continue to rise among heterosexual Americans, they are dropping among homosexuals, and educational programs have begun to affect behavior among such groups as European drug users and Kenyan prostitutes.

Traditional moral values are helpful but insufficient. Traditional moralism, however, is not helpful. We live in a society in which, traditionally, sexual activity has been supposed to be limited to marriage, and marriage was believed to be monogamous, permanent, and exclusive. Strenuous efforts were made to enforce the traditional ideals—among other things, by threats of eternal damnation. It's important to notice, as we try to adopt new kinds of guidelines for sexual behavior, that the old system never worked as it was publicly proclaimed. Adolescents have always masturbated (although they have sometimes been wracked by guilt); there has always been prostitution and illegitimacy and incest. This is discouraging, because it suggests that sexuality is so wild and powerful that even intense fear cannot control it, for our ancestors truly feared the fires of hell. Infection with AIDS is frightening, but surely not as frightening as eternal damnation. Both sickness and damnation may be long deferred, but hell goes on forever. Unlike divine justice, infection is not certain: some individuals may continue with risky behavior indefinitely without becoming infected. And yet fear of hell did not persuade the entire society to obey the rules on sex, even though fear did shape and limit their behavior and burden their consciences. This means that a lot of people have always lived by standards that diverge from those they were brought up with.

Attitudes toward the way in which behavior can be shaped have been changing. Even in many of the same denominations that once tried to motivate morality by fear, the emphasis has increasingly come to be on the love of God and the value of caring for others. Lasting changes in behavior are more readily achieved by rewards than by punishment, and sexual appetites can be channeled more easily than they can be repressed. The best way of channeling behavior toward safer sex is to find ways to make it at least as appealing as risky sex. Having a set of ideal rules about sex which are often broken is not the route to safety; it is the *reality* of sex one needs to think about.

There are always some common rules and conventions about sex that are followed by almost everyone in any group. Then on top of them there is likely to be a superstructure of ideal expectations about behavior, with

a system of built-in loopholes so that not everyone follows the ideal rules. There is not just one double standard in our tradition, suggesting that women are expected to follow the rules about sexual behavior while
men are allowed to violate them; there are many mechanisms for repairing the damage done by breaking rules
or by ignoring what has happened so that marriages can
remain intact as a means of economic and social organization in spite of violated rules. Theologically this
works; medically it doesn't. Divine forgiveness—and
human forgiveness—are both valuable in the lives of
individuals and of the community. We could use a
stronger sense of both. But it is a mistake to believe
that forgiveness makes an event "as if it never happened."
From the medical point of view, if it happened it happened. The antibodies remember.

Similarly, hypocrisy can be very useful socially. Poli-
ticians can base proposed policy for the high schools on
the ideal of abstinence from sex even while almost half
the students are becoming sexually active. They do this
not because they are stupid but because they are smart—
and more concerned about ideological advantage than
about adolescent health. This is a socially effective way
of acting that has been with us for a very long time, and
probably does provide a degree of protection and support
to those who want to live by traditional rules. Hypocrisy
is socially effective but not medically effective. Myths
influence behavior, which gives them a kind of truth.
Myths do not influence viruses.

We are having great difficulty working out new ways
of modulating sexual expression because we have spent
centuries lying to ourselves about our own sexual activity
and the activity going on around us. It's worth remembering how often in our cultural tradition we have solved
the problem of incest by punishing children for com-
plaining about it. Rules will be broken—but it is possible to have a set of rules about rule breaking that are
medically sound. Thus, even as we continue to value
monogamy, we need to understand that some departures

are more dangerous or destructive than others, just as some divorces are more caring and responsible. True lifetime monogamy is not common, since many women and most men trip up occasionally and can usually do so without destroying their marriages. We need a standard that values a particular relationship as semimonogamous and suggests that, beyond that, precautions be taken. Straying spouses could find an expression of fidelity in using condoms and not let the sense of being sinful lead to self-destructive carelessness.

The relatively late cultural elaboration of sexuality in America has had a number of costs. First, you cannot purposefully regulate or reshape an area of behavior you are determined to ignore. Neither can you enhance or enrich it. Rapid change depends on articulation. You cannot introduce conscious choice, caution, and discrimination into behavior you believe you cannot control. Gluttony emphasizes impulse, while gourmet eating emphasizes moderation and selection, for subtle flavors are lost in excess; if moderation ceased to be associated with repression, a sexual aesthetic might emerge based on subtlety and careful timing, for sometimes waiting increases pleasure. Sex for the gourmet rather than the gourmand.

In the United States, we are inclined to confuse quantity with quality. The big watery strawberries in the supermarket are tasteless compared to the fragrant smaller strawberries Europeans prefer. We are only just beginning to achieve a nuanced appreciation of sexuality comparable, say, to the Kama Sutra, and many explorations of sexuality are still tainted with lingering rage at earlier repression. As an alternative to repression and the reaction to repression, we have tended to medicalize discussions of sexuality, like so many other topics, as if an activity must be a little distasteful to be good for you—but who wants strawberries flavored with peroxide? It is now essential that individuals learn to practice and enjoy safer sex. Sex researchers are experimenting with ways to eroticize condom use and so are sophisticated men and women. Condoms are beginning to appear in porn videos as a part of foreplay rather than an interruption, and to be available in colors. The Japanese have treated condoms as sex toys for years.

When people first began discussing the dangers of AIDS it was common to refer to "safe sex," but there has been a growing awareness that safety is relative rather than absolute. It's enough to be as safe in bed with a lover as you are when riding your office elevator or flying cross-country or doing hundreds of other everyday things that carry small amounts of risk. It is a mistake to hope for a risk-free world, or to think that AIDS will soon be eliminated. But if a few individuals do contract AIDS while taking reasonable precautions, that falls in the category of being hit by a falling piano—tragic, but not a possibility you organize your life around or permit to interfere with your relationships to other people.

Safer sex suggests a range of options, with the need to discover one's own personal style. A few people may give up sex or specific sexual practices entirely; others may become very selective of partners or may involve themselves in elaborate precautions with a miscellany of plastic barriers. The bottom line, however, is the competent use of condoms, and the goal is to avoid the transfer of blood or semen from one body to the other— and to do that without giving up pleasure.

It is hard for people who know they might have been exposed to the virus not to feel a certain panic and to seek reassurance in testing, but the behavioral changes come first because they are the same regardless of the test outcome. With practice, the behavioral changes do not need to be stressful or grotesque; they can become simply routine. Panic is not the emotion that reminds you to fasten your seat belt before starting the car, or not to turn on a radio or a hair dryer on the shelf next to the bathtub, and yet in each case there are risks of death or severe injury involved. On the other hand, it is a mistake to be too sanguine. There are time delays built into the transmission of AIDS, especially where sexual activity is moderate and health is good, that can produce the illusion of invulnerability. While it is true that the level of seropositivity is still quite low outside of the risk groups that have already been identified, AIDS infection will spread in successive waves among non–drug-using heterosexuals and lesbians, and the goal is to make increased safety a matter of course before prevalence increases. Preventing AIDS is like keeping the landscape free of trash: it depends on everyone who passes through remembering never to drop a beer can or even a gum wrapper.

The guidelines that a physician would give to an individual known to be seropositive but still healthy and eager to continue an active life are the same precautions that all members of the society should be adopting in interactions with those they do not know well: a man who is infected should wear a condom during sex to prevent transmitting infection; a man who is uninfected should wear a condom to avoid contracting it; a woman should insist on male partners using condoms for one of the same two reasons. Doctors and dentists are being advised to take precautions appropriate to AIDS patients with all of their patients. Sharing hypodermic needles is always dangerous. Even in the absence of the AIDS epidemic, healthy people with no known infections should be careful with razors and toothbrushes, and should dispose of used bandages and tissues with consideration. Just as children learn to wash their hands after going to the toilet and not to borrow combs, adults need to learn to prevent transfers of blood and semen except under circumstances known to be safe. The same precautions, incidentally, offer protection from Hepatitis B, venereal disease, and other sexually transmitted diseases. Consistent condom use during vaginal, oral, or anal intercourse may not provide certainty but it is the most important step, largely protecting the receptive partner from semen and the penetrative partner from vaginal secretions, fecal material, or saliva—and both from blood and access to the bloodstream from sores and lesions.

In some ways the situation in which one person is known to be seropositive is more difficult than the situation in which either might be. The asymmetry sets up a tension in relationships with one infected partner about the appropriate expression of love. For instance, in many couples where the husband is a hemophiliac infected by factor VIII, unprotected sex continues. The wives may feel that taking precautions would be a rejection of the relationship; the husbands may feel that they are innocent casualties for whom taking precautions is an unfair penalty: "If you really loved me. . . ." These are the operative words, but who says them? The infected partner cajoling the other into risk? Or the uninfected partner remaining loyally in the relationship and preparing for a possible future of caretaking and bereavement—but not ready to convert it to a suicide pact? In such couples progression toward full-blown AIDS and infection of the spouse may not occur for years, but year by year the increments of bad news continue. People infected with the AIDS virus need to be loved and cared for—and they need to love and be careful.

Oddly enough, safer sex may mean better and more imaginative sex. Certainly it means more caring and conscious sex. In the process of discovering alternatives to penetration, there are new skills to be learned, including talking about sex with a partner and the cultivation of fantasy. Safer sex involves choice and planning ahead and a reasonable level of sobriety, lovemaking following from a thoughtful and unfuddled choice of partner—the kind one would still be glad of by daylight.

The best way to encourage responsibility is to support informed choice and to set a value on conscious decision in all actions, including conscious decisions on having children so that abortions become rare and there are no unwanted children. Planning ahead has to be associated with other desirable traits, especially for women choosing their personal styles of autonomy. Traditionally, one reason for unwanted pregnancies has been the unwillingness to admit planning for a sexual encounter—the Pill was popular because it didn't seem as specifically calculated. Couples will learn to negotiate both condom use and the trust needed for the transition to unprotected sex, often after testing or comparing histories, when a relationship begins to seem permanent or children are desired. The best stance is still the symmetrical one: both partners able to admit the possibility of exposure in the last ten years, both ready to obtain and carry condoms, and both aware that men and women often lie in the search for intimacy.

Those who are sure, because of their lifestyles, that they and their partners are safe, may feel that none of this discussion applies to them. There are a lot of advantages to a clear allegiance to traditional morality, including the protection it often offers against sexually transmitted disease, and every discussion of safer sex needs to emphasize the strengths of traditional values and the resilience and depth sometimes achieved in relationships whose exclusivity is unquestioned. Nevertheless, a few things need to be said about those who feel they are safe, particularly couples who married before the epidemic and couples in which neither partner has any previous experience. They are fortunate in that they are free to enjoy intercourse without condoms, conceiving children when they are ready or using other forms of contraception. Every member of society needs, however, to learn how to perform the basic actions of his or her life safely when others might have contracted AIDS. Just as morticians and fire fighters need to learn to take AIDS into account in their professional activities, so also do happily married, monogamous adults. Why? First, because it is better to learn how to use condoms and have safer sex under unpressured circumstances than to learn under difficult and stressful circumstances: after a spouse or lover dies, after a fluke exposure, after an incident of unfaithfulness. Competence and the skills for safe pleasure are a gift to your partner. But beyond that, adults sometimes need to be able to talk about sex with children, who ask the most unexpected questions and often sense when the answers are inauthentic. Many adults in the public health establishment talking about condom use today haven't used one for twenty years. This is understandable for bishops, but foolish for most others. There is an old joke that making love in a condom is like showering through a raincoat, but advocating condoms is often remarkably like talking through a hat.

There are other decisions that need to be made by individuals who know they are seropositive, going beyond the appropriate precautions for protecting other people. We are just beginning to understand the social and health meanings of a seropositive life, which can continue for many years, perhaps for the full expected life span, and will be experienced by growing numbers. The seropositive life is an anxious one, filled with uncertainties about personal health, the health of loved ones, and the maintenance of dignity. Anyone with an HIV infection is really afflicted by three diseases—HIV itself, personal fear, and the fear felt by others.

Someone who is seropositive may not have the combination of conditions referred to as AIDS, and may appear to be in the best of health, but he or she is infectious and faces the prospect of progression to fatal illness. A seropositive test result does not mean that death is imminent, nor does it mean the end of normal life, of love or sexual pleasure. Counseling is important not only to make clear what steps should be taken to protect one's own health and that of others, but to help individuals get the maximum benefit from the time they have—perhaps many years—rather than sink into vengeful anger or depression. Therapists who work with those suffering from terminal disease describe the process patients go through as a progression from denial through anger and on to resignation. AIDS has been defined by the medical community in such a way that the term has been applied rigorously only when the patient's condition is already effectively terminal, but for patients who are only seropositive or who have developed AIDS Related

Complex (ARC), these reactions are complicated by a mixture of hope and fear. The grief and desperation of those who know they may carry the AIDS virus include the experience of seeing friends dying from the disease, succumbing one after another to a variety of horrible deaths, and the long worry about whether to be tested.

Even though treatments are still limited, medical supervision is important. A seropositive person will watch his or her own condition with anxiety, watching for undue fatigue or unexplained sores or night sweats. He or she will also be examined and monitored by a physician to detect signs of progression to AIDS such as swollen lymph nodes, significant loss of weight, and the myriad treatable infections and tumors that afflict those with compromised immune systems. Increasing vigilance is being given to the early development of neurological symptoms, but these generally follow the development of full-blown AIDS. With time, the available clinical supports will increase. A physician or counselor can also initiate an effort to determine how the patient became infected: Does she belong to an established risk group? Has his behavior put at risk other individuals who should be contacted and advised to be tested or persuaded to modify their own behavior?

The fear felt by others is one of the most terrible burdens of AIDS infection. Everyone needs the support of other people and the nourishment of a vast number of day-to-day interactions. Studies of homelessness suggest that those who lack social networks are vulnerable to all sorts of problems, mental, legal, physical. But AIDS patients and those who carry the virus often find when they need the support of others that their social networks are severely compromised by the rejection or even terror displayed by friends and associates. Fears based on misunderstandings of how the AIDS virus is transmitted can lead to dismissal from a job or eviction from an apartment for an infected person who does not know, or is not able to fight for, his or her rights. Frequently even parents and siblings refuse their love and support, particularly if they reject the lifestyle that led to illness. Even when love and care are offered they may be compromised by inappropriate precautions, as when a mother cares for her son at home but sterilizes every utensil he uses. Doctors and nurses, afraid for their own health, may maintain a frightening degree of distance or withdraw their care in spite of their responsibility to treat and comfort. AIDS, even more than cancer, is surrounded with an almost superstitious horror, so the responses that people feel to the disease are not easily dispelled by facts. This is one reason why everyone needs to absorb the knowledge that the AIDS virus simply is not transmitted by casual contact. The reality of AIDS is devastating, but the devastation can be compounded by irrationality and fantasy.

For all these reasons, the decision of who and when to confide in about the infection is a difficult one. Someone who takes all the recommended precautions to avoid transmitting the disease is leaning over backward to avoid endangering others, so beyond these precautions there is no moral responsibility to inform them of the infection. Research shows that families live with infected individuals for many years without the disease's being transmitted, even under quite primitive conditions, and infected hemophiliac children have lived in dormitories for long periods without infecting others. It is safe to drink from the same cup as an AIDS patient, to sleep in the same bed, and even to have sex with appropriate precautions. Above all, it is safe and even essential to cradle and to comfort, to protect a lover or a child or a friend from the sense of abandonment.

Secrecy is an understandable adaptation to the disease in reaction to the risks of discrimination. The burdens of HIV infection are great enough without adding on the results of ignorance. Bad enough to discover that one's own body is freighted with death that can be transmitted to others under carefully defined circumstances, but worse by far if others mistakenly believe they can be infected by casual contact, by working together or sharing food or sitting in the same room. Secrecy brings its own kind of loneliness. It is one of the most poignant burdens on infected persons that even when they are behaving with the greatest and most responsible care, they cannot always trust others to respond rationally. Nevertheless, it is essential for those who know they are seropositive to take the risk of seeking out friends or counselors in whom they can confide fully, and to think ahead to how to prepare others to respond compassionately if illness develops. The response to the epidemic has led to the development of groups all over the country that offer friendship and social support as well as more concrete assistance.

Because the development of symptoms indicates a denser and more active viral population in the body, full-blown AIDS and ARC patients are considerably more infectious than those who are newly seropositive. But patients still healthy enough to continue normal lives should be able to do so within the same guidelines, preferably at the more cautious end of the safety spectrum. In hospitals, where blood is being drawn and unpredictable medical emergencies are confronted constantly, additional precautions for medical personnel are needed, but cherishing care by caretakers of all kinds is appropriate right up to the end.

One of the most important reasons for dealing generously with AIDS victims is so that the inevitable anger that is one of the typical reactions to the knowledge of impending death will not be turned against society. Society needs the cooperation and responsible participation of those who carry the virus, which cannot be evoked by rejection and abandonment. A supportive and caring attitude toward afflicted individuals, whatever their lifestyle or personal history, in no way conflicts with a clear condemnation of continuing irresponsibility.

Defensive measures are inevitable, but of the hundreds of AIDS-related bills introduced in state legislatures it is not easy to sort out those that are reasonable from those that might effectively increase the danger of the epidemic by undermining the capacity to cooperate against it. A number of states have already moved toward defining it as a crime for an individual who has been informed of a positive HIV diagnosis—an identified carrier—to have unprotected sex with someone unaware of that diagnosis, and justifiably so. The body of an AIDS carrier is potentially a weapon of slow death, and putting sanctions on the negligent or even deliberate use of that weapon is not an unwarranted invasion of privacy, any more than it is inappropriate to regard the fists of a boxer as potentially lethal. There are also beginning to be civil suits concerned with negligence and irresponsibility in the transmission of AIDS—for instance, in divorce cases where a wife may have been unaware of her husband's bisexuality or drug use.

There are gifts that the seropositive person cannot give without grave risk to others. Sometimes couples facing serious illness in one of the partners feel a strong need to have a child. Whatever the motivation, children born to seropositive women have a nearly 50 percent chance of a brief and painful childhood, leading to death from AIDS, coupled with the risk of growing up without one or both parents. Children conceived by uninfected women with infected partners are also at a high risk, though one can imagine the development of techniques for conception without the transmission of infection, which would permit one more dimension of fulfillment combined with loving caution. An alternative would be for healthy but infected persons to offer foster care for as long as they can to children with AIDS whose parents are already unable to care for them.

Many people find real satisfaction in giving life in another sense, by donating blood or designating their organs for use after death. It may become possible in the next few years to designate blood donations for use only in processed blood products that cannot transmit HIV, but for the present seropositive individuals, and those who know their risk is high, even if healthy and completely free of symptoms, should not donate (or sell) blood, breast milk, organs, or sperm. But here too there are alternative kinds of gifts. A substantial number of persons who realize that they are probably infected have maintained a sense of meaning and value by dedicating themselves to the care of those sicker than they, or to addressing their financial or legal problems. With AIDS, as with the common cold, it is not possible to get a second case and become twice as sick.

The decision to act in such a way that one cannot infect or become infected should be accompanied by the decision to deal with persons with AIDS as one would wish to be dealt with in that same situation. When a friend tells you he or she has AIDS, the appropriate first reaction is an embrace, not a shudder. If healthy people respond with compassion to those who have AIDS, protecting them from destitution and loneliness, those who have AIDS will be more likely to respond with the effort to protect society from the further spread of the disease.

The emphasis in this chapter has been on ways in which the kind of people likely to read this book can make responsible decisions that make them behaviorally immune to AIDS or behaviorally noncontagious. These decisions involve personal safety, the safety of partners and loved ones, and the well-being of society, for the AIDS epidemic alters forever the line between public and private morality. The precautions necessary are the same in New York and in Zaire, in Amsterdam and in Brazil, but the arguments for these decisions will have to be made again and again to fit different cultural contexts.

Not everyone has the information, the resources, or the autonomy to make such decisions. Providing these and the freedom they represent, both in our own society and internationally, is the key to social policy in the epidemic.

9

THE EPIDEMIC
AND THE SOCIETY

■

ONCE IN A WHILE, beyond the terrifying numbers projected for the future, one hears the statement that unless there are major medical breakthroughs the AIDS epidemic could bring the end of Western civilization. This is surely an exaggeration, but it is useful to clarify exactly what it might mean. Three scenarios need to be considered.

1. *Population loss*. AIDS will cause increasing numbers of casualties until the rate of spread is reversed. In the process the death rate could theoretically come to exceed the birth rate, leading to steady population shrinkage. In the countries of Africa where prevalence is highest, the population doubles in twenty-five years or less: birth rates are so high that actual shrinkage could not become a factor unless the epidemic continued unchecked for several generations. Death rates in Africa are still shaped by a whole flock of endemic diseases, and it is projected that death from AIDS could not exceed 20 percent of the total. AIDS could not solve the African population problem—but it could subvert all regional efforts to find solutions.

The demographics are different in the industrialized countries, where general health factors probably ensure slower spread in the non–drug-using heterosexual population; but within specific communities they may be worse, and the demographic impact of AIDS will be sharpest in the great cities that are also our cultural centers. The end of civilization is not going to come about through simple loss of population due to the AIDS virus. Arguably, indeed, Europe benefited from the Black Death, which hastened the decay of medieval institutions and opened the way for the Renaissance. AIDS is similar to warfare in that the toll is highest on those in the prime of life; but functioning societies can recover remarkably quickly from massive population losses, and there are good reasons why epidemics tend to be self-limiting, as this one will surely prove to be. Diseases are rarely uniformly lethal, so the portions of the population that survive are those with natural resistance of some kind. We do not yet know for certain whether there are individuals whose own immune systems can withstand or resist HIV infection indefinitely, but there probably are. In addition, AIDS presents the possibility of behavioral immunity: anyone can make the decision to be immune by avoiding high-risk behavior, and many follow traditional patterns that already protect them. Societies have choices of how to respond, however, that may affect them long after demographic perturbations are over.

2. *Resource depletion*. AIDS will cause major economic disruption and painful choices in resource allocation which might cripple a given society or make it vulnerable to other kinds of attack. Health care costs are already a source of economic instability in the United States and the care of a single AIDS patient approaches $100,000, while the number of patients is increasing steadily. As the resources of more and more individuals are drained, more of this will become a public charge, adding to deficits. The carefully planned profitability of the health insurance industry is threatened—and so is the belief that any private industry can solve public problems like those of health care with a modicum of fairness. There will be needs for personnel and hospital facilities as well,

needs that might prove to be transient. Money spent on AIDS may increase public deficits or force hard choices of taxation or reductions in other expenditures. Because the sums will be so large, major decisions of priorities will be needed. It will not be sufficient to reallocate available funds within the category of public health or human services.

This is a problem that may appear to weigh more heavily on affluent societies, where expected standards of health care are very high, than on the less developed countries, but that contrast is delusory. Officials of the United Nations Children's Fund point out that the epidemic will cause the death of more children through the diversion of resources from other public health programs than will die of AIDS. It is important to consider the cost of what does *not* happen because of the epidemic, such as the lost earnings and participation of those who die in the prime of life and opportunities missed. The AIDS epidemic may be the final straw for societies unable to establish self-sustaining economies.

In the developed world, the economic threat of AIDS will cause a certain amount of disruption in some industries and profit in others. The problem comes as always in decision making: What is the public priority on easing the pains of the dying? What are the relative values of therapy and prevention? How important is research on the immune system's defense of the body compared to research on space defense? Both will benefit basic science and have massive spinoffs, but different groups of individuals will draw the primary profit. How about drug interdiction and the immense profits of the illicit drug industry?

The concept of *triage* is a way of thinking about resource allocation on matters of life and death that originated on the battlefield. The nurse at the emergency room desk, who makes decisions about the order in which patients are seen or the need to call additional help, is called a triage nurse because of her role in sorting out need in relation to resources, but the term goes back to situations in which resources were so scarce that some patients could not be treated at all. On the battlefield, the wounded were divided into three groups: those who were so severely wounded that they would probably die even if treatment were given, those whose wounds were so slight that they would recover without treatment, and those for whom treatment would make the difference between recovery and death. In real scarcity, the third group must take priority, but we live in an affluent society that expects to be able to provide the convenience and reassurance of care for many who probably don't need it, as well as offering heroic measures for those who are close to death. AIDS is going to put major strains on resources, however, and it seems certain that new standards of care for patients with brief life expectancies will develop, including appropriate levels of intervention that will be applied to cancer patients and to the very old.

In principle, triage is ethical when it reflects real limitations and is consistently applied, but it can easily be converted, even in the emergency room, into a form of discrimination based on ideas of differences in human worth. Still, redefinitions of appropriate care can lead to improved care as well as to the withdrawal of care. Many people with only a few months left of life would prefer to spend the time peacefully becoming used to the approach of death rather than undergoing one violation after another. The AIDS epidemic could lead to improved home care, improved hospice care, and improved psychological support for the dying. It could also confirm and extend in us habits of treating groups as expendable and callously ignoring human suffering.

The AIDS epidemic will amplify the effect of past choices and priorities, and the choices we make now will leave a continuing mark on society. The adverse effect of AIDS on the economy will be more a matter of ill-chosen priorities and bad planning than of direct costs.

3. AIDS will cause *psychological and social reactions that may change the character of human social life*. If the epidemic

were to induce us to give up travel or international communication or were to sabotage our tenuous capacity for global cooperation, it would quite literally be undermining civilization. It also has the potential for creating political instability in third world societies where public order is already precarious, particularly in cities, and such instability can spread.

More narrowly, if reactions to the epidemic compromise basic values too pervasively, the epidemic could destroy the more recent and potentially more vulnerable institutions of democracy. If AIDS drives us into coercive and repressive social policies, it will have tempted us away from the basic commitments of our society. It could benefit society for individuals to become more aware and selective in their sexual practices, but a wave of puritanism or repression would work against creativity. Like the Black Death in Europe, AIDS could trigger religious movements embracing ignorance, massive scapegoating, or paranoia, a failure of hope or of compassion. It could in a generation subvert the fragile structures of dedication in the medical profession.

It is this third kind of danger, danger to the way society is organized, that is the basic threat of the AIDS epidemic. Thus it is that a consideration of how to respond to the AIDS epidemic directs us back to our own values. Our view is that many ways of reacting that might be effective would represent a compromise of those values, but that if those values were more effectively realized, our danger would be reduced. The AIDS epidemic cannot help but be a source not only of self-knowledge but also of self-determination, a way of understanding the choices that make us who we are and clarifying our priorities as a society. Just as it is possible to ask what the characteristics were of gay liberation in the 1970s that made the gay community so effective in amplifying the epidemic, so it is possible to ask about the characteristics of national policy in the 1980s that have made it so difficult to respond, and about the characteristics of a future society able to deal with the disease. The society must respond to the epidemic while maintaining basic constancies—that is, without compromising identity or fundamental value commitments. This capacity can be thought of as the immune system of society.

There are real choices to be made at a national level, choices that reflect quite different premises about human beings. So far, responses have been inconsistent, reflecting sometimes one way of thinking and sometimes another. Different national styles have been clearly visible: the Swedes displaying huge posters of condoms in the streets and the United States avoiding even the word on television, the Soviets deporting seropositive foreign students and some developing countries denying that the disease even exists. Even New York and California have shown visibly different cultural styles, while national policy has fluctuated and waffled.

It is possible to argue that there are two contrasting ways of dealing with the epidemic, each of which might be successful, each of which would leave its mark on the societies that adopted it.

On the one hand, it is possible to respond to the epidemic by reaching for a more open, just, and intercommunicating society and world in which no one is disenfranchised and individuals have the information to make appropriate decisions. Thus if we were able, as a society, to talk openly about matters related to sex and to feel compassion equally for all of our neighbors, the AIDS epidemic would probably be under control by now. Instead, we are in a situation where help has been withheld because of unstated ideas about who is and is not deserving, where essential information is not imparted to those who need it, and where many lack the trust and self-esteem needed to use the information available to them. The perennial problems of our society and of the world, which we have not had the resolution or imagination to address, are the principal source of vulnerability.

It is clear that the disease proliferated first in populations that have every reason to suspect they will be treated unfairly, and that the existence of prejudice is the main continuing barrier to communication. Homosexuality, extramarital sex, and I-V drug use are still stigmatized as antisocial or sinful behaviors by many, and the health problems that accompany them are sometimes seen as divine punishment. The same residues of prejudice give others a false sense of security. Racial and other minorities are sensitive to the possible "good riddance!" of the larger society and justifiably sensitive to the possibility that those who have discriminated against them for so long will find the epidemic a good excuse to do so again. The epidemic flourishes on discrimination and exclusion. Furthermore, stigmatized populations are burdened by a partial acceptance of external views. "Internalized homophobia," and "low self-esteem" make individuals value their own lives and health less, leave them with less hope for the future.

Internationally, the unequal distribution of resources and concern creates the setting for the proliferation of the disease. If health care in central Africa were comparable to that in industrial societies and part of a worldwide communicating network on the lines of the U.S. Centers for Disease Control, the epidemic might have been stemmed at a local level. In a genuinely interconnected and intercommunicating world, monitoring of health problems must be international. On the other hand, it is hard to imagine an effective shift in health delivery systems without substantive changes in other conditions, including the conditions that make so many people dependent on a living earned in migratory labor. There is no way of knowing for sure where the epidemic originated, but we do know that African populations suffer so many scourges that a new disease can proliferate unseen. The entire planet is vulnerable when certain areas are neglected.

Nationally and internationally, disease and drug use thrive on poverty and inequality. In America, the epidemic developed in a period when government was withdrawing from social programs, cutting budgets in all nonmilitary areas, and using the machinery of regulation to promote economic productivity rather than individual welfare. Disease also thrives on ignorance. Programs to control the spread of HIV can be blocked by unwillingness to talk candidly about sex. How many deaths will result from the refusal to use the word *condom* on television? Reluctance to use the word *semen* apparently led to the unfortunate euphemism *bodily fluids*, which escalated public anxiety by suggesting that HIV is likely to be transmitted by sweat or saliva or tears in casual and domestic contact. People have been driven from their homes as a result of such artificially maintained ignorance.

Each of the issues mentioned here is connected to other severe social problems, ranging from famine in Africa to teenage pregnancy to the increase in homelessness and malnutrition that accompanied government withdrawal from supporting social programs. The notion that affluence will spread through the society from the privileged to the underprivileged is called the "trickle-down theory." The reality that the result of allowing the AIDS epidemic to develop among marginalized groups will be its spread into the mainstream might be called the "trickle-up theory."

But this is the liberal point of view, the belief that social problems can be addressed by education and that behavior can be improved by equity. An alternative point of view would reflect other kinds of social agendas: If the society had more effective control over sexual and other private behavior, perhaps it could simply prevent promiscuity. If the concern for human rights had not been so expanded, it would be possible to deal with the epidemic by isolating it, to test everyone and intern all carriers, extruding them from society as was once done with lepers. If we were not burdened by concern for individual welfare there would be no need to struggle to prolong life for those already infected, no high insurance costs, no painful decisions about schooling. If police powers were expanded, borders could be effectively closed, drug traffic interdicted, and traffickers shot. It does indeed seem probable that the epidemic would be easier to deal with if we were a less open and caring society. Compassion can be expensive, and certainly the costs of the epidemic are increased by the desire to alleviate suffering. So far, the Soviet bloc seems to be less affected than the West, and Islamic fundamentalism does provide a model for one way of reducing homosexuality and other kinds of sexual activity: by treating them as capital crimes.

In general, there is a mirror-image quality to the costs and benefits of particular social institutions. The blood bank industry and the bathhouse industry both resist regulation within the ideology of capitalism, and the Bill of Rights protects beliefs we deplore as well as those we adhere to, allowing both information and misinformation to spread.

Against this background, we believe that policies based on openness and equity have the best chance of success, providing a framework for policy recommendations for reacting to the epidemic domestically and internationally. The proposals that will be made here are idealistic in their goals, but this is because of our conviction that survival under threat must mean the maintenance of the basic premises of the society, premises that have a certain biological as well as social logic. These proposals are not based on the assumption of universal altruism, but rather on the assumption that we as a society can recognize this as a situation in which the general welfare benefits from care for individuals and from empowering individuals to care for each other.

Policy must be thought through place by place. There are tasks to be done in every school and corporation, every town and city. AIDS policy is often treated like a hot potato, passed from person to person and from agency to agency. More painfully, individuals with AIDS are often routed from place to place or hospital to hospital, even deported from country to country. Because the private challenges of developing a personal behavioral immunity to AIDS must be faced everywhere, it is necessary that the public challenges be faced consistently, so that the visible institutions of society support molecular change. The following, then, are some of the places where change is needed.

■

IN THE SCHOOLS AND COMMUNICATIONS MEDIA. The handling of sex education represents a major philosophical inconsistency in American society: the belief that the social good is best achieved by enforcing ignorance of possible options rather than by informed choice. There are many who are more comfortable with that way of doing things. Recent lawsuits brought by some fundamentalist groups about textbooks have protested against any stimulation of the imagination through fairy tales and mythology as well as exposure to different belief systems and aspects of scientific knowledge. There is also an inconsistency in the argument that children can be exposed to violence and weapons with impunity, but will be corrupted by exposure to information about sexuality. Furthermore, the ignorance we conserve is never total. Children not taught about sex pick up misinformation from their classmates. We cannot afford to conserve ignorance about sex. The alternative is to present it so early that it is clear that the information is not an invitation to immediate action.

The management of the classroom has always been important in public health education, alongside actual lessons. Particularly in the lower grades, children pick up ideas of nutrition and sanitation from school practices like hand washing and discarding dropped food and the reactions when a child is hurt. School management should be based on the possible presence of students who are knowingly or unknowingly seropositive, and this in itself is an important lesson for adult living.

Once we manage to clarify what knowledge is necessary for a responsible adaptation to a world that contains the AIDS virus, and once a commitment is made to information in preference to ignorance, it follows that the media should provide specific and candid information and corrections to misinformation—and this should take precedence over considerations of taste. The effort will be long, and hard to maintain in focus. Much can be done by including safer sex in story lines, just as smoking has been progressively excluded and interracial casts have become routine.

IN THE WORKPLACE. It is the task of all managers and all those making administrative decisions on the organization of work to maintain a workplace in which transmission of infection is prevented—part of a general effort to maintain health and prevent industrial accidents—and to be sure that misinformation does not lead to discrimination. No one should lose his or her job because of false beliefs about how AIDS is transmitted. Similarly, no qualified person should be denied a fair chance for a job because of the possibility of developing AIDS—this is comparable to refusing to employ women because they may eventually have children. No employer welcomes the complexities of dealing with disability but no equitable hiring policy can avoid it. An open and matter-of-fact policy toward the disease and the distribution of information are ways of promoting realistic prevention. Discrimination goes with magical thinking about one's own safety.

IN THE STREETS. There are two issues here. First, America cannot afford to maintain an underclass that is chronically impoverished and alienated. The despair of unemployed youth in the ghettos often leads directly to I-V drug use, but it should be addressed in its own right, not because it promotes the spread of AIDS. Treatment should be easily available for all addicts, with the possibility of methadone support and even govern-

ment-supplied heroin and hygienically run public shooting galleries. Addicts should not have to rent needles
because carrying their own might lead to arrest. But
these are half measures unless people are given alternatives: quality education, real access to employment, reason to aspire toward the future. Even the classic escape
of the disinherited through the armed forces is now often
closed, as the military services become increasingly selective. We need to offer every girl and boy a life that
is more attractive than drug addiction.

Similar arguments apply to prostitution, which has
been a major factor in the spread of AIDS in Africa and
will probably be increasingly important elsewhere. The
sex industry resembles I-V drug use in that you cannot
make something safe if you pretend it isn't there. Many
countries, such as the Netherlands, regulate prostitution
and carefully supervise health in order to control venereal
disease. Again, this is a necessary first step, but it needs
to be combined with programs that will increase the
options available to women in the sex industry, many of
whom are also afflicted with problems of low self-esteem
and many of whom have been long-term victims of
exploitation and molestation. "The world's oldest profession" is not likely to go away, but women who choose
to remain in it could benefit from better control of their
own conditions of work, just as addicts who remain
addicted are better off with safer and cheaper drugs.

Second, America cannot afford the massive enrichment
of drug dealers and their destructive effect on the lives
of youth. Drugs are a multimillion-dollar international
industry so large that it threatens political stability in
many regions of Latin America. There are estimated to
be over a million intravenous drug users in the United
States, which was a tragedy of major proportions before
AIDS, contributing to a whole range of other social
problems. In some cities, 60 to 80 percent of heroin
users are already seropositive, and here the group that is
perhaps hardest to contact and persuade has to be persuaded to change both sexual and needle-sharing behav-

ior. The largest numbers of infants born with AIDS are the children of this population, largely black and Hispanic.

Many proposals to make the drug-using population more accessible involve partial decriminalization of some kinds of drug abuse. The criminalization of any behavior creates the motivation to support it and makes it difficult to reach those who are involved. Whatever hesitations we might have about the government supporting drug addiction or the sale of sexual services are minor compared to the cost of criminalization. In fact much of the pressure against partial or complete decriminalization of many crimes probably comes from those who see the connection between profitability and illegality.

■

IN THE DRUGSTORE. Someone should design a hypodermic needle that cannot—mechanically—be reused, and it should be available as cheaply and easily as Kleenex. Failing that, handy portable bottles of bleach solution for cleaning needles and syringes are needed. Condoms are another product that should be available as cheaply and easily as Kleenex, not only in stores but in vending machines in multiple locations and along with the free shampoo in hotel rooms.

■

IN THE MARRIAGE OFFICE. Gay rights provide the best path to gay responsibility. We need both. We need to create an environment that is accepting and supportive of gays precisely so that they will feel like full members and participants in the society, with all the responsibilities that entails. You cannot selectively approve and disapprove aspects of someone's behavior by starting from a blanket condemnation. We cannot expect those with homosexual preferences to fit into social expectations of sustained relationships unless we treat gay and lesbian relationships as equivalent in value to heterosexual relationships. Marriage is hard enough to maintain in a society that approves of it and values it. This would mean finding ways to register and celebrate new commitments, permitting gay couples to adopt, preventing discrimination in housing, and treating same-sex companions as legal spouses. Saint Paul was speaking of heterosexual marriage when he said that it is better to marry than to burn. There seems to be no question that the voluntary concentration of gays in a few urban neighborhoods has provided a breeding ground for disease, but it would be reduced if gays were not made to feel uncomfortable elsewhere. We know that the gay community has produced many of the heroes of the epidemic so far, and men who were at one time involved in impersonal sex have nursed their loves selflessly while others have given all their resources to help the community, setting extraordinary examples for the rest of the society.

Stable relationships are valuable to society for many reasons, not just to prevent the spread of AIDS, and this means that all policies and legislation that work against them should be altered. This is especially true of welfare, since the need for welfare often forces couples to live separately and drives them apart.

■

IN THE CLINIC AND THE WARD. Policy toward those who are actually sick should deal with individuals in ways that express society's value commitments and elicit their cooperation and trust. This will mean changes in society's response to illness of all kinds, not only to AIDS, which will involve public expenditures and more flexible policies. One common form of medical discrimination practiced implicitly in our society is to give more and better care to people who are felt to have no responsibility for their diseases, and this kind of inequality needs to be addressed. It will not be acceptable, however, to make massive diversions of health funding, and so it seems likely that the AIDS epidemic will cause a long-overdue rethinking of the American health system. This may involve some reductions in available health care, for there is certain to be a demand for controlling medical costs by reducing heroic medical interventions at public expense that will make no more than a few days' or weeks' difference, and if this is implemented throughout the system without discrimination, it seems reasonable. Experience in the AIDS ward of San Francisco's General Hospital suggests that when patients are in an environment where they are deeply convinced that every effort is being made to sustain quality of life, there is less insistence on futile and expensive interventions.

Although many patients live for considerable periods—even several years—after developing Kaposi sarcoma, and many recover from a bout of Pneumocystis pneumonia and are able to lead normal lives, there comes a time when multiple opportunistic infections converge and medications begin to conflict, a final slide toward death. Fortunately, there is a gradually emerging ethic, represented by the hospice and home care movements, that values making that final period as peaceful and comfortable as possible. It is not reasonable to expect the society to subsidize forms of care that are regarded as ineffectual. This applies to all patients, not just AIDS patients. It is unethical to prescribe massive doses of medication or expensive treatments to support the illusion of activity.

Individuals with full-blown AIDS will make choices that, while not putting other people at risk, are widely disapproved of, and here there seems to be a great deal to be gained from tolerance. Some will pursue therapies that the medical profession regards as valueless but that the victim experiences as helpful. Some will wish to commit suicide, and are being helped to do so responsibly in some European countries. Logically, it makes sense to try to dissuade individuals from suicide after a first diagnosis, when a considerable period of nearly normal living is still available without risk to others, but this epidemic may become the occasion for a reconsideration of the individual's right to end his or her own life. Voluntary euthanasia probably promotes more careful consideration and even postponement than the need some feel to achieve suicide before they become incapable of independent action, trapped in a hospital bed, and some suicidal improvisations are dangerous to others or lead to costly and unwanted emergency procedures. Because so many victims are at the prime of life, AIDS will probably be the focal point of thinking about death and dying over the next decade, and all Americans may be the beneficiaries of the increased sensitivity and realism it engenders.

AIDS patients also differ from other groups close to death in their concern for self-determination, including making their own decisions on treatment. Currently this is leading to a form of guerrilla medicine, unsupervised self-care and experimentation with unproved therapies. The solution is a greater partnership and respect between providers and patients, including respect of patient acceptance of experimentation and risk.

Hospital administrations will have to deal with fears of infection in their personnel. The numbers suggest that these fears are very much affected by public hysteria. There are 6.8 million people working in health care, and so far there have been nine cases of AIDS directly attributable to occupational accidents, occurring mostly when recommended precautions were not being observed. Hospital administrations have a two-sided task: at the same time that they must make sure health care workers do not neglect AIDS patients, they need to persuade workers actually to observe standard precautions. Supporting the morale of health care workers and protecting them from burnout and the impact of repeated failure will also increase willingness to work with AIDS patients.

Another kind of publicly supported medical investment is needed for better care of conditions that are not life-threatening but can be co-factors of AIDS, including all of the sexually transmitted diseases.

■

IN THE RESEARCH LAB. Medical research and drug approval will also call for restructuring. There is a demand for relaxing some of the restrictions on experimental drugs and permitting their use with patients who are clearly terminal. AIDS-related research is of many different kinds. The search for a vaccine has been immensely popular among drug companies but offers less promise of controlling the epidemic than do education and social change—there are huge theoretical and delivery problems to be surmounted before AIDS could go the way of smallpox and polio. The very concept of vaccine may be inapplicable because of HIV's use of the immune system itself. However, only medical research and treatment can address the problems of those actually infected with the virus, controlling or ending its ravages, treating opportunistic infections, and ultimately reconstituting the immune system. There are also issues about the coordination of research, since in some areas close coordination is most useful while in others a thousand flowers should bloom. Perhaps secrecy and duplications of effort motivated by the desire for a Nobel Prize or for huge manufacturing profits should be regarded as opportunistic infections of AIDS research, but the scientific community seems to do much of its most creative work under the spur of competition.

■

Implementation of policies like those just discussed is necessarily a piecemeal process, with decisions and procedures being taken at hundreds of different points. But human behavior is not generated piecemeal; rather, it expresses basic premises carried from one context to another and specifics learned by analogy. The best way to persuade individuals to behave differently in the bedroom is to create a consistent climate that is expressed in those more public places that are more easily influenced by public policy: in the classroom and in the boardroom, on the street corner and on the evening news.

Each of these proposals addresses an area where individual decisions are not likely to be adequate and public policy making is needed, but each needs to be complemented by new kinds of caution in all groups, personal decisions balanced and supported by public commitment. The same general principles hold, however, for both public and private behavior: responsible choices rest on genuine freedom; fear is a poor teacher; delay means loss of lives. If the population at large does not alter its sexual behavior until it has experienced the depth of loss and direct contact with suffering that the gay community has experienced, it will be too late to change.

■

Can we then visualize a society voluntarily arrived at in which all drug addicts and prostitutes are reformed and responsible members of society, all teenagers are cautious about sex, and all gays are semi-monogamous? Of course not. The vision here is of a society in which these choices are genuinely accessible, supported, and valued, and, because the choices are open, more aspects of behavior will be accessible to influence. But there is no such thing as a society in which every member is responsible.

Each of these proposals, phrased here in relation to the United States, needs rethinking and rephrasing to make it applicable in other parts of the world. It seems clear that any measures that combat ignorance and illiteracy and poverty will be helpful if the basic thrust is to give people genuine choice in protecting their own lives. AIDS drives home the message of global interdependence and demonstrates that sharp differences in quality of life are a source of instability. At the same time, rather basic information about the dangers of infection can make a difference in behavior, provided the individual has a sense of having choices. Those who are addicted to drugs feel that they have no choice; those who can barely buy food will not pay for condoms; those who do not know the alternatives cannot choose among them. The AIDS epidemic proposes a new commitment at a global level to literacy and economic opportunity.

It will not happen overnight. The first goal is a society in which the epidemic will cease to spread, and this means a society in which on the average each person infected with AIDS will transmit the disease to no more than one other person, over an apparently healthy infectious lifetime of five years or more. The next step must be to force the epidemic to recede. The number of people with full-blown AIDS will continue to rise for a decade unless there are major medical breakthroughs, and will level off five to ten years after the rate of new infection levels off. The rate of transmission per infected person has probably begun to slow, but the numbers of new infections are still rising.

What about costs? Every one of the proposals mentioned here requires social investment that will save money later. We live in a society that spends money lavishly on military preparedness under the rubric of "defense," but in this situation we should read a new meaning into that term. Talk about epidemics is always full of metaphors from warfare, metaphors of invasion and defense and infiltration, and in the area of expenditure at least, a military metaphor is useful. The most useful model for the kind of scientific mobilization needed to combat the AIDS epidemic may be the Manhattan Project. The most useful model for the social response to the epidemic is surely the response of urban Londoners to the Blitz: defense based on calm realism and mutual concern.

Outside the economic area, these warlike metaphors are flawed by the same simple assumption of competition that pervades most evolutionary discussion. Once in a while it is reasonable to speak of the total defeat of a disease, as in the eradication of smallpox. More often, the task of public health is an adjustment of mutual boundaries and niches that lowers the toll of disease. It may be that ultimately it will be possible to defeat AIDS. But in the meantime, it should be possible to learn to live with AIDS—possibly, indeed, to live better.

Warfare is an activity with only a single purpose, an activity in which priorities are simplified and energies are focused on a single goal of victory. But the proposals laid out here have multiple goals. Safer sex can control most sexual transmission of disease, and provide an effective option of family planning to whole populations. A genuine effort to improve conditions for minorities can bring all the benefits of full social participation, flowing in both directions. AIDS is a powerful reminder that ignorance and injustice are themselves insidious diseases that endanger the entire world community.

10

AFTERWORD

■

As LONG AS AIDS was a mysterious and unexplained plague, it could be seen as something separate from human society, an act of God or of random chance or of uncaring nature. But now that we understand its mechanisms—not a mysterious plague but an intelligible epidemic—it has become subject to human decision and social policy. Important as it is to work for medical breakthroughs, the epidemic could be halted entirely by social means, either by means appropriate to a pluralistic society or by means that are coercive and draconian. Either could be effective; either would affect the character of those who used them. When the time comes to count the cost of the epidemic, it will be counted not only in lives lost and dollars spent but in the effect it has had on our institutions and on our understanding of the human condition. This is a way of saying that the threat to society has to do with politics and value systems as well as demographics and economics. At the same time, society might benefit in many ways from lessons learned in these areas.

The basic approach of this book has been an exploration of what it means to be a species shaped by both biology and culture. On the one hand, we are the product of genetic information and the influence of natural environments. On the other hand, we pass information from one person to another and from one generation to another, learning to shape our environments. In the control of the AIDS virus, we can hope that the transmission of knowledge will prove to be more effective than the transmission of infection.

It would be a mistake, given the diversity of ethical conclusions reached by different human groups, to claim to derive ethics directly from biology. Experience suggests that human beings tend to perceive the natural world in terms of their social experiences rather than vice versa, rewriting natural history to justify capitalism or communism, hierarchy and male dominance or co-operation, imperialism or pluralism. Nevertheless, it is still useful to look, at times of choice, for possible congruence. It is our conviction that an exploration of the distinctive adaptations of our species can suggest ways of looking at the epidemic, and that a metaphorical movement between biology and culture is one way of seeking consistency.

The social experience that the West brings to meet the biological threat of disease is one of democratic pluralism inconsistently maintained and called into question again and again by what are presented as imperatives of biology. It is our conviction that the appropriate responses to the epidemic are in fact congruent with democratic traditions, and that there is guidance to be found in the consistent application of pluralism and democracy. In effect, we are arguing that concern for individuals and open communication are good biology.

In the historic crisis created by the AIDS epidemic, we are dealing with a confrontation between life forms with diametrically different evolutionary strategies. The AIDS virus is an example of minimum structure, rudimentary functioning, and rapid variation. Each individual virion is utterly expendable, for at the microbial end of the evolutionary scale, adaptation is served by heavy and rapid selection in organisms sufficiently simple so that random mutation is relatively likely to propose viable possibilities. Microbes, insects, and most invertebrates are spendthrift of progeny, counting success in the survival of a tiny fraction of the offspring produced. Many are born, and most are wasted.

Human beings are at the opposite end of the scale. Our ethical intuitions of the value of the individual are congruent with our biology, for each human individual, and above all each individual reaching maturity, represents a very great investment for the species. The entire description of the immune system in chapter 3 can be read as a parable of commitment to individual survival, for except among a relatively few vertebrate species, safety is in numbers and each individual is undefended against infection. Even in preindustrial societies, over a third of the infants born alive survive to reproduce. The rearing of those infants requires not one or two years of care, which are relatively common periods in other large mammals, but ten to fifteen years, for humans are born almost totally helpless and achieve true viability only after years of learning and loving care. Few are born, and few are wasted.

Paradoxically, we have become so successful that the planet is overburdened with these precious progeny, but this does not change the human capacity to value individuals. We still respond to individual tragedy in the face of vast numbers, and understand increasingly that the path of wisdom is to limit births and dedicate ourselves to optimizing the chances of each individual born. The value of the human individual is a fact of evolutionary strategy; the capacity to care for individuals—at least for our own children—is essential to species survival. Even when all actual child care is done by the mother, she depends on the support of others and on a community. Human survival has depended on cooperation rather than simple competition.

Before suggesting that there is a biological basis for the value of the individual, one should consider the alternative. It could be that the human species would benefit from drastic pruning, that we would be better off for a pandemic that eliminated half or more of the planet's burden of human beings. Perhaps, it has been said, those with genetic predispositions to drug addiction will be weeded out, homosexuality or perhaps promiscuity in general will be eliminated, and the continent least able to feed its population will be freed from famine. Perhaps for once the ignorant and feckless will not be rewarded with the greater progeny, but instead the world will be populated by the children of those who restrain their impulses and plan ahead. And all of this could be achieved without concentration camps, but only by "letting nature take its course."

These are arguments that are being made in many quarters. There are those who take the extreme view that the slowness of the U.S. government in responding to the AIDS epidemic was not a matter of blindness and ineptitude but a deliberate passivity that has been called passive genocide. Why indeed struggle to preserve the lives of "junkies and perverts"? Why, more broadly, do we invest so much in the preservation of individual lives, painstakingly separating Siamese twins, grafting skin on burn victims, and transplanting organs?

Why has a concern for individual human lives emerged as so important for human society that it outweighs the benefits of natural selection? Perhaps because a concern for individuals and for the development of diverse individual potentials has been a necessary theme in the shift from biological to cultural evolution. Now that we depend on cultural evolution, we have to ask what kinds of societies provide maximum scope for the emergence of original thinking. What kind of society can muster the skill and intelligence and teamwork to unravel the mysteries of the immune system? Only one in which individual talent and diversity are valued and brought into interaction.

A similar set of arguments can be made for the congruence between certain kinds of communication and basic human patterns of adaptation. Because we survive by knowledge, we flourish in a knowledge-rich environment. We are only just beginning to know how to run societies so that the talents and capabilities of all members can be tapped. It is clear that a strategy for dealing with the AIDS epidemic through knowledge and communication highlights problems in our present communications environment. Too many people do not believe what they are told—perhaps with reason. Too many in fact cannot read. Here, too, there are implications for contemporary society.

These issues converge in yet another important fact about human adaptation: the continuing value for human communities of those individuals who do not or cannot reproduce but can communicate. Human beings tend to outlive their reproductive capacities, but the oldest members of any community are often treasured for their wisdom, for what they have to say. Similarly, societies have flourished in which large numbers of those who were most talented had no physical progeny but became, for reasons of asceticism or sexual preference, artists and thinkers and conservers of the general good, sustainers and builders of civilization.

Just as the values of communication and concern for individuals are congruent with the human pattern of adaptation, so also is a recognition of the unity of our species and the interdependence of different species in the environment. Willingness to care for individuals within the family or community has not always been extended to other groups, even to those close at hand. When the poet John Donne wrote that he was diminished by each single human death, there were still multiple human populations on this planet unknown to each other and unlinked for millennia. Today that is no longer true. We have all heard the terrifying remark that when we make love, we are intimately linked to every partner our lover has slept with in a ten-year period and to those partners' partners, linked back in a ramifying network of shared passion. We may know our partner and our partner's partners, but two or three links away in the chain there are intimacies in different worlds of experience, down streets we would never walk or even on other continents. Indeed, the AIDS epidemic is the shadow image of the multiple networks of interaction that now unite our species. The hyperbole of infection, even though it is an imagery of horror rather than beauty, is reminiscent of the blue-green image of the earth seen from the moon, defying all borders and divisions projected upon her, united by atmosphere and oceans into a single living community. The most serious dangers that threaten her, including the dangers of overpopulation and pollution, are far more difficult to address than the AIDS epidemic.

We are obliged to act from the sense of being a part of a larger whole: in the words of the microbiologist René Dubos, who projected an ethical vision derived from his knowledge of living systems, we can address the crisis only by "thinking globally and acting locally," choosing patterns of responsible behavior and struggling to offer freedom to make the same choices to those who are constrained by ignorance or poverty or addiction. We can protect ourselves only by protecting others and sharing what we know.

SUGGESTIONS FOR
FURTHER READING

■

ALTHOUGH AIDS is a recent development, its literature is already vast. At this writing more than 100 books and in excess of 10,000 research papers addressing some aspect of AIDS have been published. Those who try to enter this lush jungle of print without some notion of the paths to take will find that they have entered a truly bewildering landscape. To help those who want more information to guide their thinking about AIDS, we offer a purposely short list of readings and a word about where to look for new developments.

First, for coverage of what's new and newsworthy in relation to AIDS across-the-board, from sociology, economics, and politics to virology, immunology, and medicine, the New York *Times* catches most of it. Those who want more detailed and rigorous coverage of medical and technical issues will want to turn to such flagship journals of medical reportage as *The Journal of the American Medical Association*, *The New England Journal of Medicine*, and the premier weeklies of scientific research, *Science* and *Nature*. Those who are intrepid in their pursuit of the developing epidemiological picture of AIDS will want to look at the *Morbidity and Mortality Weekly Report* (*MMWR*), a dry-as-dust current status report on the epidemiology, diagnosis, and occasionally therapy of many diseases, including AIDS, published by the Centers for Disease Control, the U.S. Public Health Service's superb monitor of the nation's health.

For the best summaries of current knowledge, the following articles are suggested: "The surgeon general's report on acquired immune deficiency syndrome" was published in *The Journal of the American Medical Association* 256 (1986): 2784–89. With a terse, no-nonsense eloquence, the U.S. government made it official: AIDS is important. This document also contains some hard-headed advice on risks and how to avoid HIV infection. Read this along with: "Revision of the CDC surveillance case definition for acquired immunodeficiency syndrome," *Morbidity and Mortality Weekly Report* 36, supp. #1S (1987): 1–15, the detailed and surprisingly clear medical definition. The virological background is described in R. C. Gallo, "The first human retrovirus," in *Scientific American* (December 1986): 88–98, and "The AIDS virus," *Scientific American* (January 1987): 47–56. Together this pair of articles by a pioneering researcher in the field provides a lucid and fascinating introduction to these deadly engines of disease.

Medical aspects are reviewed in "AIDS: What is now known," a series of four articles written by Peter A. Selwyn, M.D., for *Hospital Practice*, a respected medical digest, as a primer on AIDS for doctors. If you have a medical dictionary by the reading table, these articles are accessible to the layperson who is curious to know what doctors are telling each other about this disease. The papers are:

1. "History and immunovirology" (May 15, 1986): 67–82.

2. "Epidemiology" (June 15, 1986): 127–64.

3. "Clinical aspects" (September 15, 1986): 119–53.

4. "Psychosocial aspects, treatment prospects" (October 15, 1986).

Another state-of-the-art compendium appeared in a special *Science* issue (February 5, 1988; vol. 239) that included eight articles on several aspects of AIDS, each prepared by an individual or a group particularly well placed to have a definitive view of their area.

1. P. Piot et al., "AIDS: An international perspective," pp. 573–79.

2. B. M. Dickens, "Legal rights and duties in an AIDS epidemic," pp. 580–86.

3. R. W. Price, et al., "The brain in AIDS," pp. 586–92.

4. H. V. Fineberg, "Education to prevent AIDS: Prospects and obstacles," pp. 592–96.

5. L. Walters, "Ethical issues in the prevention and treatment of HIV infection and AIDS," pp. 597–603.

6. D. E. Bloom and G. Carliner, "The economic impact of AIDS in the United States," pp. 604–10.

7. J. W. Curran et al., "Epidemiology of HIV infection and AIDS in the United States," pp. 610–16.

8. A. S. Fauci, "The human immunodeficiency virus: Infectivity and mechanisms of pathogenesis," pp. 617–22.

One last biomedical presentation is a book-length compendium of articles: *Aids: Facts and Issues*, edited by Victor Gong and Norman Rudnick (New Brunswick, NJ: Rutgers University Press, 1986).

By the time the items on this list have been digested, new ones will have appeared, but there are a few books that will not go out of date. One of the best places to start is with *The Plague* by Albert Camus (New York: Alfred A. Knopf, 1948). This extraordinary novel of a North African town besieged by an epidemic has come to be recognized as a prescient parable of human reactions to AIDS. As a correction for the tendency to infuse the biological phenomena of disease with too much meaning, we recommend *Illness As Metaphor* by Susan Sontag (New York: Farrar, Straus & Giroux, 1978), a sharp lens of a book that helps one see through and cope with the historic tendency of society to confuse and conflate certain diseases with matters moral or aesthetic. The actual narrative of the history and the evolving politics of the epidemic up to 1987 is presented by Randy Shilts, an impassioned and sharp-eyed journalist from San Francisco, in *And the Band Played On* (New York: St. Martin's Press, 1987).

INDEX

■